What people are ~~saying about~~

Grandma's Drugstore Treasury...

I really enjoyed reading this wonderful book. It was very informative. I think you have an excellent resource here to pass along to many through the ages. You deserve all the awards and some more too. Everything is so easy to gain access to. **~Paul Frey, author**

A friend sent me your book and I think it's great. I have a page of my grandmother's recipe's on my first ever site. Your book is fabulous and unique. **~Margaret (Margie) Hayes**

Great Old Recipes! **~Susan, Suisan City, California**

WOW! Great, great, great! Can you send me about 10 more? I've got people in mind that need to read this before the New Year. **~Leah, Jacksonville, Florida**

Your book is delightful. Very interesting and entertaining. Thanks for sharing. **~Carole, Goodyear, Arizona**

I cannot begin to tell you how very much I have enjoyed this book! It is so easy to see that a lot of thought, effort and love have gone into creating it and making it the best book I have ever read on holistic health and treatments. You are so kind to share these remedies with all of us and so much appreciated. Although I work in the Base Hospital where different methods are used for ailments, I am going to recommend this site to my supervisor, as she too believes that there are at times alternative methods in treating non threatening ailments. Many thanks for all that you have done to make this book what it is, perfect in every way! **~Lynn, Biloxi, MS**

Thank you. I enjoyed this book very much and plan on buying several more for my daughters. (Maybe they'll learn a thing or two). **~Pat, Fort Edward, New York**

I've really enjoyed reading your cures! I can't wait to try them! **~Patti, Glendale, Arizona**

Love your entries. I am constantly buying books on home remedies. I think that yours may be next on my list to reorder as gifts. **~Christie, Alexandria, VA**

Thanks, Shawna!! It came out great!! God bless you! **~Donna**

This is one of the best books I have ever read! **~Diane, Kent, WA**

This book is fantastic. It is bookmarked for many rereads and uses! **~Brenda, Cape May Court House, NJ**

This is the greatest!!!! **~Pat, Westminster, CA**

I've never done this before, that I was so impressed with a book that I had to E-mail the person to let them know what a great book it truly is. I had been looking for home remedies and was fortunate enough to come across your website. Great site, fantastic book. Keep up the terrific work. **~J.M. in Seattle**

What a great thing to stumble upon. With two year olds I have a lot of ailments and I do NOT feel comfortable giving lots of medicine. I am very glad to at least have the 27 to try out at home. By the way do you know of anything that will stop two year olds from biting and spitting???? :) **~Danielle, Mesa, AZ**

I have to say that this is by far the best and most unique book that I have ever encountered. It's great and very informative. Thanks! **~Cyndee, Pinellas Park, FL**

Just wanted to write and let you know that I love your book. Keep up the good work! **~Benji**

LOVE YOUR BOOK. Please let me know when you come out with another. **~Judy, Anaheim, CA**

This is better than *Chicken Soup for the Soul*---and a lot more fun and usable! **~Janice, Las Vegas, Nevada**

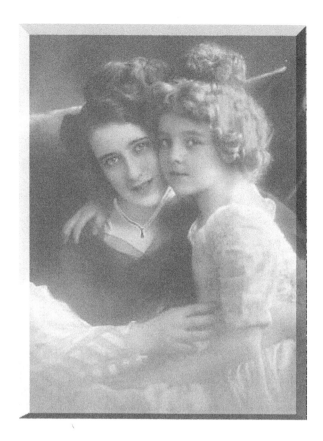

Disclaimer

I had wanted to write this book for years. The desire began with my own interest in having one book with these remedies right at my fingertips for my own personal and family's use. That was a dream, and I soon began research to find "tried and true" home remedies from women's journals. I own over 30 books on herbs, natural healing and beauty, along with countless notes taken from historical books and old publications bought at garage sales. Additionally, there were the stacks upon stacks of notes from "grandmothers" I talked to in the past.

The research for this book has been exhausting, yet fun. The problem I kept running into was that if I or a friend needed a certain remedy that used ingredients readily at hand in the kitchen, I would have to go through all the written works I had collected to locate it. Finding a specific remedy could be time-consuming, tedious, and frustrating---especially when there was an ailing child, wailing in the background who, obviously, COULDN'T WAIT ONE MORE MINUTE to get relief.

I have not gone into an abundance of detail about the attributes of the different herbs and ingredients used in the remedies. That was not the purpose of this book. However, I have listed several herbs and their uses in "Introduction to Your Kitchen Cupboard" along with additional herbal references in the back of the book.

If you however, would like to have more information in this area, there are many informative books on herbs at your local library, bookstore, or health food store. Part of my goal while writing this book was to: include only the recipes that use ingredients that are probably already in your kitchen cupboard or easily and inexpensively obtained from a drug or grocery store.

Please bear in mind that herbs are MEDICINE. Never use them in place of your doctor if there is any question of a serious condition. The recipes in the Health section, especially, are intended to be used for GENERAL SYMPTOMS OR AILMENTS. While many, many herbs are currently being used safely as foundations for some prescribed medications for more serious conditions, it is wise to be prudent.

MOST herbs are safe when used in the specified amounts. SOME herbs do not work well with, or counteract, properties in a prescribed medication. ALL herbs should be respected in their own right. NEVER abuse them.

Many of the remedies and recipes contained in Grandma's Drugstore are also comprised of various foodstuffs.

When in doubt, always ask a physician, pharmacist, or expert herbalist.

The author does not accept liability for use of the recipes/remedies. While most of the ingredients are safe, it is wise to consult your physician if there is any doubt of possible effects if herbs are used in conjunction with other drugs, or if certain other allergy/medical problems exist.

Please review the information at the back of the book for food and herbal interactions.

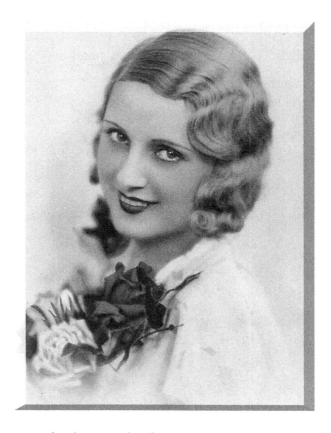

Acknowledgements

Special thanks go to my husband Michael Newton, for his patience in being a "writer's widower" while I was compiling this treasury---on three different occasions, no less: 1992, 1996, and 2008.

I would also like to thank my aunt, Diane Buchholz, who has been supportive with her love, guidance, and suggestions for editing. She is one of those spirits who "walks her talk" and I am blessed to have her in my life. Thank you, Auntie.

I would be sorely amiss if I did not also thank the Grandmothers who recorded their recipes in journals for the next generations of Daughters. I hope that they and their families have smiled upon my efforts to bring their remedies into a culminated work for all to enjoy in this sometimes-discouraging age.

I wish I could acknowledge and thank each of them personally; however, many of their writings were unsigned. Let it suffice that everyone who reads this book will in some way, lovingly reflect on these women who have gone before us. These women were the health and beauty advisors and experts of their day, and desired to pass on their "recipes" and wisdom by writing them down in journals.

There is a reason "Grand" precedes "Mother."

May all the Daughters of today appreciate and remember why this is so.

Shawna Nero Newton, September 22, 2008

Grandma's Drugstore is

Dedicated To

Norv and Lynn Nero,
without whose support, guidance and love,
I would never have known the value and beauty of
individuality, creativity, and perseverance.

ISBN   978-0-557-01885-7

Preface

The First Edition of Grandma's Drugstore was completed February 22, 1996. In the beginning, I took my 8 ½" x 11" manuscript to Kinko's and ran copies. With our technological advances through the years, I had later turned the manuscript into a digital book.

Today, Grandma's Drugstore is in hard copy. So many people have requested a paperback version of the book through the years, I am sure this book will be granting some wishes.

The inspiration for Grandma's Drugstore came from my great-grandmother, Augusta Glawe. As a child, I knew that no matter what happened, "Gukkie" had a way to fix any situation. Much of her wisdom came from her previous years in nursing but more often than not, she used the Power of Prayer.

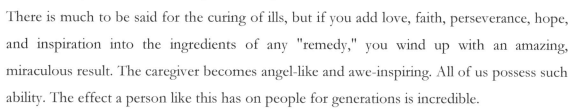

Therefore, Grandma's Drugstore is inspired by Augusta Glawe, a.k.a. "Gukkie," and the reader will find several of my personal "Gukkie Stories" scattered throughout these pages.

Healing is an art that can be learned. Augusta Glawe, affectionately called "Gukkie" by her family, was a born healer. There is much to be said for the curing of ills, but if you add love, faith, perseverance, hope, and inspiration into the ingredients of any "remedy," you wind up with an amazing, miraculous result. The caregiver becomes angel-like and awe-inspiring. All of us possess such ability. The effect a person like this has on people for generations is incredible.

I know that I would not be the person I am today without having had her influence in my life. You would not be reading this book, either. Thus begins her story...

At an early age in her life, Gukkie was drawn to helping others. She inherited many of the old German ways of her mother. To my knowledge, Gukkie's mother (my great-great grandmother), ran a tight ship with her brood of eight children. In fact, one story is told about how, in her last days, Gukkie's mother, over 100 years old, embroidered pretty flower designs on her bed sheets. This busy-ness was an attribute that passed on to Gukkie.

At 16, Gukkie became a nurse for the town doctor. The technical knowledge was not her primary goal. She found this to be an area where she could be a positive as well as healing force in the lives of others. Her medical education was an added benefit, not the first, to the men, women, and children she ministered.

Gukkie's nursing career ran off and on during the years. Her expertise in the medical field served to act as a life boat when she needed to earn a living. This became no more apparent than when she became a widow at an early age. After the sudden and early death of her husband she found herself in serious debt. Almost all her possessions were liquidated in order to clear those accounts. She found herself with almost no money at all and two children to support on her own. Therefore, the nurse in her sprang into action and Gukkie enlisted in the Women's Army Air Corps (WACS) during World War II.

Taking her fun and loving spirit with her, instead of resentment of her life's circumstances, Gukkie began the "healer's service" in and out of uniform throughout her many years ahead. Gukkie could not only treat a cold, but treat the heart as well. Always.

Without such giving of herself to bring out the best in other people, her remedies would be missing a prime ingredient that knocked out the cause of any ailment. This prime ingredient was true love and concern for humanity. Because of this, Gukkie touched the lives and warmed the hearts of literally hundreds of people during her lifetime. As you will see by the stories throughout this book, Gukkie is someone you will come to know and love. You will also learn by her examples, and her methods of "treatment". One cannot simply have the ingredients to any remedy without the method of preparation and administration---with love.

Hers is a story that never ends; the giving of herself continues to perpetuate itself as a living entity throughout the years after her passing. Hers is a personality you want in your life. Her walk is one many struggle to emulate and attempt to achieve with the same extraordinary results.

Through these pages, you are going to get to know her. And if your life is touched by something you read in one of her stories, Gukkie would smile.

And maybe an Angel would sing.

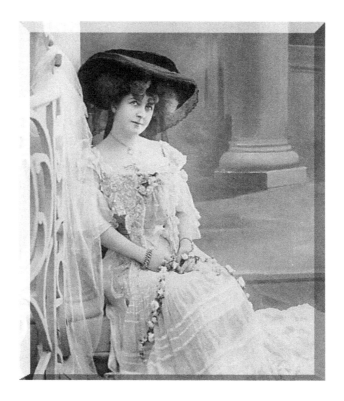

Table of Contents

Introduction to Your Kitchen Cupboard

You will find many remedies and recipes that contain the same ingredients. Many herbs are so strong and versatile that they fit the bill for many different kinds of purposes. Some of these favorites are:

Aloe Vera – Healing

Baking Soda - Neutralizes Acids

Borax – Cleanses

Castor Oil – Fixative

Cider Vinegar - Ph balance and Antiseptic

Cornstarch - Healing and Soothing

Epsom Salts - Soothing and Muscle Relaxing

Garlic - Antiseptic and Antibiotic

Gelatin – Protein

Ginger - Antiseptic and Antibiotic

Glycerin - Moisture-Retainer

Honey - Antiseptic and Antibiotic

Lemon - Kills Bacteria

Mineral Oil - Non-Spoiling Oil

Oatmeal - Cleansing and Soothing

Olive Oil - Premium Oil

Onion - Antiseptic and Antibiotic

Plain Yogurt - Easily Absorbed and Healing

Sage - Antiseptic and Antibiotic

Salt - Astringent and Antiseptic

Vitamin C – Preservative

Vitamin E – Healing

Wheat Germ Oil – Healing

Witch Hazel - Astringent

ACNE & BLEMISHES

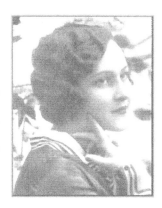

BAKING SODA

Make a paste of baking soda and water. Apply to the face and leave on for 5 minutes. Rinse off with hot water with 2 Tbs. apple cider vinegar in it. Rinse again with clear water. Apply a coating of vitamin E oil to your face and leave on overnight.

BASIL

For acne that hasn't seemed to respond to anything: Use 2-3 tsp. dried basil leaves to 1 cup boiling water. Steep 10-20 minutes. Cool, and apply with cotton ball.

BICARBONATE OF SODA

Rub blackheads with a solution of bicarbonate of soda and distilled water.

BORAX

1 Tb. of borax to 1/2 pint of water is an excellent remedy for cutaneous eruptions (pimples).

BROWN OR YELLOW LAUNDRY SOAP

Applied to pimples will bring them to a head, or even dry them up. This treatment is also an excellent remedy for boils.

BURDOCK

Burdock is an exceptional astringent, removing excess oil from the skin. Use it faithfully every day if your skin is oily. It may take several weeks before you notice an improvement. Put 2 handfuls of burdock roots and leaves in 2 cups of water. Bring to a quick boil using a stainless steel or glass pot. Lower heat and simmer 10 minutes. Dip clean cloth into liquid and use as a compress until the cloth cools. Repeat this, keeping the liquid hot, for about 15 minutes.

BUTTERMILK

Apply buttermilk to skin and allow to dry for about 10 minutes. Rinse off with cool water to close large pores.

CHAMOMILE

Boil water and add it to chamomile flowers. Make an umbrella "hood" with a large towel. Cover your head with the hood, keeping your eyes closed. Allow the chamomile steam to open the pores of your face. Cleanse face immediately afterward. Embedded dirt and blackheads will be easy to wash away.

CUCUMBER, CORIANDER AND MINT JUICE

A teaspoon of coriander juice, mixed with a pinch of turmeric powder, is another effective home remedy for pimples and blackheads. The mixture should be applied to the face after thoroughly washing it every night before retiring. Mint juice can be used in a similar manner as coriander juice. Grated cucumber applied over the face, eyes, and neck for 15 to 20 minutes has been found effective. This tonic is wonderful for the skin of the face. Its regular use prevents pimples and blackheads.

FENUGREEK

Fenugreek is another useful remedy for acne. A paste made of the leaves of this vegetable, applied over the face every night before going to bed and washed with warm water in the morning, prevents pimples and blackheads.

GARLIC

Garlic has been used successfully in the treatment of acne. Pimples disappear without scars when rubbed with raw garlic several times a day. Even extremely persistent forms of acne, suffered by some adults, have been healed with this herb. The external use of garlic helps to clear the skin of spots, pimples and boils. The process is further helped by eating three pods of raw garlic once daily for a month to purify the blood stream, so as to secure a long-term clearance of the skin.

JUICE

Ginger juice

1/4 inch ginger

4 - 5 carrots

1/2 apple, seeded

Extract the juice from the above ingredients, mix well. Apart from being an effective detoxifier, ginger also freshens up ones skin as it is a good source of zinc.

Dose: Take 25 ml per day

LANOLIN, GLYCERIN, & CASTOR OIL

Mix equal parts and melt this concoction over low heat, let it cool and keep it in a GLASS jar. Apply to pimples until healed.

LEMON

Rub lemon juice on blackheads around the nose. Lemon has also proved beneficial in reducing pimples and acne. Its juice should be applied regularly to obtain relief

OATMEAL, WHITE WINE & LEMON JUICE

Cooked oatmeal mixed with white wine and lemon juice and left on the face overnight gently forces blackheads out and closes pores.

ONIONS

Cook an onion in lard until transparent. Allow to cool, and place between pieces of cheesecloth as a poultice. Helps heal pimples and blemishes.

ONION JUICE

Clean face thoroughly. Apply fresh onion juice to the area. Leave on for 15 minutes. Rinse well. Use daily.

ORANGE PEEL

Orange peel has been found very effective in the local treatment of acne. Pounded well with water on a piece of stone, the peel should be applied to the affected areas.

PARSLEY

Put a large handful of chopped parsley into an earthenware bowl. Pour 1 cup of boiling water over parsley. Cover and let steep until room temperature. Strain and apply the liquid to the face as a compress for about 15 minutes. Use daily. This mixture unclogs pores and clears up the complexion.

STRAWBERRIES

Rub the face with a crushed strawberry. Leave it on for about 15 minutes. Rinse thoroughly with warm, then cold water. This will help to clear blemishes. Caution: Many people are allergic to strawberries. Try a patch test before proceeding to use the facial treatment.

THYME

Because thyme is such a good astringent, it can be used to help clear up acne. Pour 1 1/2 cups of boiling water over 3-4 tablespoons of dried thyme. Let steep 30 minutes. Strain and bottle the liquid. Keep refrigerated. Teenagers with acne problems could use this daily as a facial rinse.

VINEGAR

Add 1/2 to 1 cup apple cider vinegar to a basin full of very hot water.

Rinse face several times for optimum Ph restoration.

VITAMINS

Two vitamins, namely, niacin and vitamin A have been used successfully to treat acne. Vitamin therapy should comprise the intake of 100 mg niacin, three times daily, and 50,000 international units of vitamin A, three times daily. Vitamin E, 400 mg, should be taken once daily. This therapy should be continued for a month.

ZINC

Another effective remedy in the area of nutrition that seems to offer new promise of help for acne is zinc. Zinc has shown dramatic results in some cases. Zinc should be taken in therapeutic doses of 50 mg three times a day. Zinc is available in tablet and in capsule form. The patient can take a dose of 50 mg daily up to one month or till there is noticeable improvement and then reduce the dose to 25 mg.

GUKKIE AND HER SUITCASE

Gukkie's suitcase didn't contain only clothes. Her suitcase was a treasure trove of mysterious goodies; fabric, sewing notions, bottles of stuff, and packages with undiscovered contents; her bible was always on top.

My dad used to tease her about how the suitcase weighed a ton. He knew. He had to carry it. After picking Gukkie up at the airport when she visited, she would find something to giggle about all the way home. I never saw her mad or cry. I'm sure she did but she hid things like that.

She prayed the bad things in life away.

The first thing I had to do after hugging her was to wait until she got ready to unpack the suitcase. I'd sit there and try not to be too noticeable about staring at it while the adults took their sweet time catching up on all the latest goings-on in the family. I just knew Gukkie had something special in that suitcase for me, and there always was. It was usually something she had made, and most of the time it was a doll or stuffed animal. Whatever she made I clung to until it fell apart or grew so old that it would fall apart if my mother washed it one more time.

However, most of the time, she brought things to put together to fill the needs of other people. If she knew my mom needed drapes, she had her sewing kit and often, the very fabric my mom was looking for. On the other hand, if someone was feeling under the weather, hosts of remedies were in the lining of the suitcase. You just never knew what could be there but you could bet she read people's minds as well as their hearts.

Most people pack the things they need when they go somewhere. Their suitcase contains only what they need. Some things just never change. Like the '70's, "I, I, I, Me, Me, Me" way of thinking.

Why is this?

Many, if not most teenagers today think that way---as well as their parents. Somehow the notion of "when you fill a need in someone else besides yourself, you feel so good" got lost in "what's in it for me?"

It's a shame when people do not recognize that part of making life worth living is in giving.

If people re-discovered how good the giving of themselves made them feel, we would not have the drug and alcohol problems we have today.

Gukkie was always "high" on life in all of its true reality.

She knew how to pack her suitcase no matter where life took her.

BATHS

BICARBONATE OF SODA & PERFUME OR ESSENTIAL OIL

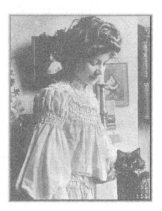

For bath salts, take 5 oz. soda and a few drops of your favorite oil. Pound and mix all the ingredients well and keep them in a decorative closed jar. Dissolve a handful of salts in the bath water before stepping in.

LIQUID DISH DETERGENT, UNFLAVORED GELATIN, GLYCERIN & EGG

For a bath full of long-lasting bubbles (a Gukkie favorite), combine 1/2 c. dish detergent, 2 packets of gelatin, 1 Tb. glycerin, and 1 egg white, and stir well until mixed well. Pour under running water.

OATMEAL, VANILLA EXTRACT & BAKING SODA

Combine 1 c. oatmeal, 1 c. warm water, 1 Tb. vanilla extract, and 1/2 c. baking soda in a blender or food processor until you have a smooth paste. Pour this paste under the running water while drawing the bath. Very soothing to dry, itchy skin.

PINE NEEDLES

Place 1 c. pine needles in a large pot on the stove and cover with 2 c. water. Bring the water to a boil and remove the pan from the heat. Allow the pine water to cool, about 30 minutes., then strain off the needles and discard. Pour the remaining water into a clean bottle. Add to bath water for a gentle and relaxing bath.

BAKING SODA, & EPSOM SALTS

Mix 1 c. of each and pour into the filling bath slowly, allowing the mineral to dissolve completely. This mixture is very relaxing and helps after an especially hard day.

WILD THYME, MARJORAM & COARSE SALT

Take equal parts of each, place into cheesecloth or muslin and tie. Place in bath for a wonderful aroma and relaxing experience.

Massage Oils for After Bath

LIGHT OIL, CINNAMON, & VANILLA EXTRACT

Mix 1/2 c. oil, 1/2 tsp. cinnamon, and 1/2 tsp. vanilla extract. Let sit for several hours. Strain into bottle. Men love this one.

ALMOND OIL & CORNSTARCH

Mix 1/2 tsp. of both extracts, 1 tsp. of the almond oil. Place 1 c. cornstarch in resealable bag or container. Add the oil mixture, seal container, and shake gently until all the powder is mixed.

PEPPERMINT OIL, VODKA & CORNSTARCH

Mix 1/2 tsp. of the oil and 1 tsp. vodka. Place 1 c. cornstarch in container. Add the oil and vodka and shake until the powder is mixed. VERY refreshing.

CITRUS & OIL

For an exciting and uplifting massage, pace 1/2 c. assorted citrus zest (yellow part only of peel) into a glass or ceramic bowl. Pour heated oil over the zest and heat.

DANDRUFF & HAIR GROWTH

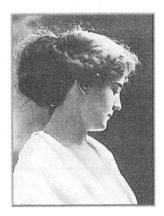

APPLE CIDER VINEGAR

The vinegar is poured into the hair, massaged into the scalp, and left to dry for a few minutes. Then the hair is washed. The process is repeated daily until the dandruff disappears, usually within a few days.

APPLE CIDER VINEGAR & MINT LEAVES

For a dandruff rinse, place 1/2 c. apple cider vinegar and 1/2 c. fresh or 1 Tb. dried mint leaves in a ceramic bowl. Pour 1 c. boiling water over mixture, allow cooling completely, and then straining out the mint leaves. Apply to scalp as a final rinse after shampooing. Finish with a cool, fresh-water rinse.

ASPIRIN

Dissolve 10 aspirins (5 grains each) in 1 cup warm water. Massage into scalp for about 10 minutes. Rinse thoroughly. Add a vinegar rinse as an extra help after rinsing aspirin out completely. Use after every shampoo as needed.

BEET

Beets have been found useful in dandruff. Both tops and roots should be boiled in water and this water should be massaged into the scalp with the finger tips every night. White beet is better for this purpose.

BURDOCK DANDRUFF TREATMENT

In a separate container, mix 1 cup burdock, 1 cup peach tree leaves, 1 cup chamomile, 1/2 cup sage leaves. Pour 8 cups of cider vinegar into a gallon jar. Add the herb mixture to the cider vinegar. Let stand for 2 weeks. Strain and apply morning and evening. Do not rinse off. Let dry on hair. Wait until the next day to rinse it out. There is no need to use any soap or shampoo to rinse out the treatment. Using plain water will wash this treatment along with the dirt from your hair. This works quickly on dandruff. To darken the hair with this recipe, add 1 cup of hop flowers to the herbs before allowing them to steep in the vinegar.

CASTOR OIL

Rub castor oil into scalp and swallow in a small amount to encourage hair growth and give it extra shine.

DRIED NETTLE DANDRUFF TREATMENT

Add 4 tablespoons of dried nettle to 2 cups boiling water. Steep overnight. Strain and add 1 cup of apple cider vinegar. Massage into the scalp. Can also be used as a face rinse to get rid of oily skin. Apple cider vinegar is great to use for scalp treatments, facial treatments, or simply to add to your bath. It helps to keep the skin clear if you drink a little vinegar water a couple times a week. Add honey, and you will keep your whole body toned up.

FENUGREEK SEEDS

The use of fenugreek seeds is one of the most important remedies in the treatment of dandruff. Two tablespoons of these seeds should be soaked overnight in water and ground into a fine paste in the morning. This paste should be applied all over the scalp and left for half an hour. The hair should then be washed thoroughly.

GINGER

To increase blood circulation and nourish hair roots to encourage hair growth, finely grate a chunk of ginger. Warm it slightly, spread it on the bald area, cover it with a shower cap or plastic wrap for 30 minutes. Wash off. Do not use if this recipe if the skin is broken on the scalp.

HONEY, VODKA, & ONION

For balding, mix 1 Tb. of honey, 1 shot of vodka, and the juice of 1 onion. The combination is rubbed into the scalp every night, covered, then rinsed off in the morning.

JALAPENO PEPPER, VODKA, & CASTOR OIL

To stimulate hair growth, chop 2 small or 1 large pepper into tiny pieces and place in small glass or ceramic bowl. Pour 1/2 c. vodka over peppers and allow to sit for several days.

Strain off vodka and discard peppers. Add 2 Tb. castor oil, mix well, and pour into bottle. Shake before using. Massage a small amount into scalp before going to bed. A slight tingling sensation will be felt on the scalp.

LIME

The use of a teaspoon of fresh lime juice for the last rinse while washing the hair, is another useful remedy. This not only leaves the hair glowing but also removes stickiness and prevents dandruff.

OLIVE OIL & ASPIRIN

For dandruff control, combine 10 crushed aspirin in 1/2 c. olive oil and mix well. Massage mixture into scalp for 2-3 minutes. then leave on scalp an additional 5 minutes. Rinse well with cool water for at least 1 min., then shampoo as usual.

ONION

For baldness, rub a little onion juice on your head and lie out in the sun.

PARSLEY

This is a great rinse and helps to control dandruff too. Pour 2 cups of boiling water over 1/2 cup of chopped parsley. Let stand 30 minutes. Massage into scalp and allow to stay on 15 minutes. Use as a final rinse.

ROSEMARY, GLYCERIN & COLOGNE

For dandruff, take 3 Tbs. Borax, 3 oz. rosemary, and steep mixture in 1 qt. of boiling water. When cold, add 1/2 oz. glycerin and 30 drops of cologne. If the hair be moist or oily, use 1 Tb. or borax in a 2-3 times weekly shampoo.

ROSEMARY & OLIVE OIL

To stimulate hair growth, mix 2 Tb. dried rosemary and 1/2 c. olive oil. Heat but do not boil. Cool completely and let sit for 2-3 days, then filter out all the solids. Massage a small amount into scalp after shampooing and before going to bed.

OTHER REMEDIES

Dandruff can be removed by massaging the hair for half an hour with curd which has been kept in the open for three days. Another measure which helps to counteract dandruff is to dilute cider vinegar with an equal quantity of water and dab this on to the hair with cotton wool in-between shampooing. Cider vinegar added to the final rinsing water after shampooing also helps to disperse dandruff.

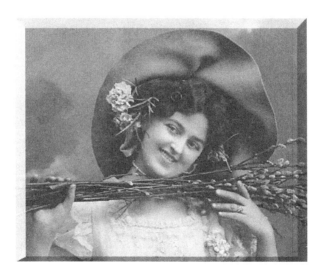

FACIALS, MASKS, & TONERS

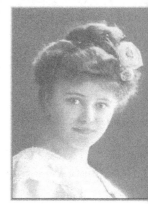

AVOCADO & BANANA

Mix 1/2 average-size mashed avocado and 1/2 mashed ripe banana together until smooth and creamy. Spread on face and leave on for 15 minutes. Rinse. Perfect for dry skin.

BUTTERMILK & POWDERED MILK

Mix 1/4 c. buttermilk and 1/4 c. powdered milk to form a smooth paste. Spread on an even layer of paste over face and neck. Let dry 15 minutes. Rinse with cool water. Store in refrigerator. Makes skin smooth and glowing.

CARAWAY

Grind or crush 1 tsp. of seeds, and steep in 1 c. of boiling water. Drink as a tea to bring color to the cheeks.

CARROT & MAYONNAISE

Mix 1/4 c. grated carrot with 1 1/2 tsp. mayonnaise. Spread on face and leave on for 15 minutes. Rinse. Carrots hydrate the skin and help clear away dead skin cells.

COGNAC (OR ANY ALCOHOL), EGG, NONFAT DRY MILK POWDER, & LEMON

Mix 1 Tb. alcohol, 1 egg, 1/4 c. milk powder, and the juice of 1 lemon in a blender, or stir well with a wire whisk. Apply to face and allow to dry, about 15 minutes. Rinse. Store in refrigerator. Moisturize afterward.

CUCUMBER

Massage the face with fresh cucumber slices. Cucumbers have a cooling effect on the skin and eyelids.

DRIED APRICOTS, NONFAT DRY MILK POWDER & HONEY

Blend 1/2 c. dried apricots, 1/2 c. warm water, 1 Tb. milk powder, and 1 Tb. honey in blender and blend until smooth. Spread on face and leave on 15 minutes. Rinse. Revitalizes complexion.

MINT & APPLE CIDER VINEGAR

Mix 1 Tb dried mint leaves or 3 Tbs. fresh to 2 Tb. vinegar and 1 C. distilled water. Stir thoroughly and allow to sit for 3 days. Strain out the mint leaves, and use a cotton ball to apply to face.

OATMEAL & BUTTERMILK OR EGG

Mix a little oatmeal with buttermilk or the white of an egg, and spread it liberally on your face. Allow at least 20 minutes for the mask to dry and draw before rinsing off. Follow up with an herbal steam facial for extra effect.

OATMEAL, EGG, LEMON, & APPLE

For oily skin, mix 1/2 c. cooked oatmeal, 1 egg white, 1 Tb. lemon juice, and 1/2 c. mashed apple into a smooth paste. Apply to face and leave on 15 minutes. Rinse.

OATMEAL, EGG, BANANA, & HONEY

For dry skin, mix 1/2 c. cooked oatmeal, 1 egg yolk, 1/2 mashed banana, and 1 Tb. honey to form a smooth paste. Apply to face and leave on 15 minutes. Rinse.

ROSEMARY

Soak rosemary leaves in white wine and use as a hand and facial wash. Perk up a complexion with a steam facial made with rosemary leaves.

UNFLAVORED GELATIN & FRUIT JUICE

Combine 1 packet gelatin (about 1 Tb.) and 1/2 c. fruit juice in glass container. Heat gently to dissolve gelatin completely. Put in refrigerator and cool until almost set (about 30 minutes.). Spread a thin layer over face and allow to dry. Peel off, and rinse face with cool water. Refreshing.

VITAMIN C & LEMON

For a quick pick-me-up and freshener, dissolve the vitamin C tablet in 2 c. boiling water. Place yellow part of 2 lemons in a ceramic or glass bowl and pour the water/vitamin C mixture over it. Let sit for several hours. Remove peel and pour remaining liquid into a spray bottle. Used to rehydrate skin and hair.

VODKA, FENNEL, & HONEY

Combine 2 Tb. vodka, 1 Tb. fennel seeds, and 1 1/2 tsp. honey. Stir well and allow to sit for 3 days. Strain mixture. Use full strength or add 2 Tb. water to dilute. Use a cotton ball to apply to face as a toner. This was also a tried and true recipe for wrinkles. (And I have tried this one and can vouch for its effectiveness...I love it...).

HAIR CONDITIONERS & RINSES

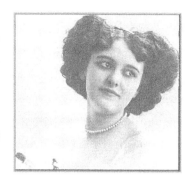

BAKING SODA

To remove build-up from gels and hairsprays, combine 1 Tb. and 1 c. water to use as a rinse.

CANTALOUPE

For a light conditioner for oily hair, take 1/2 c. mashed cantaloupe and massage into hair before or after shampooing. Leave on 10 minutes. Rinse with cool water.

CASTOR OIL

Rub into scalp and swallow in small amounts to make hair grow rapidly and give it extra shine.

CIDER VINEGAR

For brown-haired people, add 4 Tbs. vinegar to three glasses of water. Massage the mixture gently through the hair and rinse with cool, clear water to remove the vinegar odor. Adds highlights. For blonde-haired people, use only white vinegar.

EGG

A nourishing conditioner for dry or damaged hair which can be used for all hair types: Separate the white of an egg from the yolk, whip it to a peak. Add 1 Tb. of water to the yolk and blend until the mixture is creamy. Then mix the white and yolk together. Wet your hair with warm water, remove the excess moisture, and apply the mixture to your scalp with your fingertips. Massage gently until the froth is worked into your scalp, then rinse the hair with cool water. Keep applying the mixture until it is used up and then rinsed until all the egg is washed away.

FLOUR

Mix 1 c. flour and 1 c. water until you have the consistency of batter. Apply to dry hair before shampooing. Leave on 10-20 minutes. Rinse hair with cool water until all the paste is removed. This could take 5-10 minutes. (Do not use hot water.) Shampoo and rinse well. This recipe makes hair EXTREMELY SHINY.

HONEY OR MOLASSES

For blondes, use 1/2 c. honey and massage into hair. Leave on 20-30 minutes. Cover with plastic wrap. Brunettes use molasses in the same manner, as molasses will not lighten the hair.

LEMON JUICE, VINEGAR & BEER

Any of these, used as a rinse, seals in moisture and seals dirt out. Increases hair fullness and avoids tangles. Use equal parts of water to the lemon juice, vinegar, or beer.

RUM & EGG

For body and shine, mix 3 Tb. rum and 1 egg. After shampooing, pour mixture into the hair and leave it in for 1-2 minutes. Rinse with very cool water.

TOMATO JUICE

Use 1 c. tomato juice after shampooing to remove odors in the hair, such as smoke. Use a tepid rinse.

UNFLAVORED GELATIN, EGG & LEMON

For smooth and shiny hair, dissolve 1 packet (or 1 Tb.) gelatin in 1/4 c. warm water. Stir well. Add 1 egg and 2 Tb. fresh lemon juice. Shampoo hair, apply mixture and leave in for 1-2 minutes. Rinse with warm water, followed by a cool rinse.

HAIR DYES & HIGHLIGHTERS

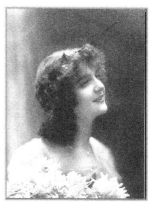

BAY RUM, OLIVE OIL, & BRANDY

To color human hair black and not stain the skin, it is asserted that a liquid may be made by taking one part of by rum, three parts of olive oil and one part of good brandy by measure. The hair must be washed with the mixture every morning and in a short time the use of it will make the hair a beautiful black without injuring it in the least. The articles must be of the best quality mixed in a bottle and always shaken before use.

CHAMOMILE

To bring out the highlights in blonde hair, use 3 to 4 Tbs. of dried flowers to a pint of water. Boil for 20-30 minutes. Strain when cool. Hair should be shampooed before rinse is applied as hair must be free from all oil. Apply rinse and brush through. The application may be repeated; brushing and rinsing.

COFFEE

Strong, black coffee makes an excellent hair dye for brunettes. Pour cooled coffee over head, and wait 20 minutes. Rinse out the coffee with beer, vinegar, or lemon juice to seal in the color. Finally rinse your hair with clear water.

LEMON

For blondes, take the juice of two lemons strained through cheesecloth and mix with an equal amount of lukewarm water. If possible, leave this solution in your hair and let it dry in the sun. If you do which to rinse it out, use cool water.

POTATO

For blondes, pare a dozen potatoes, cover them with cold water and let them boil in an iron pot until soft. Strain the water off and leave it to cool, being careful that it touches nothing, lest it stain. Make a thorough application of it to the hair and then in order to set the color, let the hair dry in the sun.

RHUBARB

To lighten hair, use 1/4 c. chopped fresh rhubarb to 2 c. boiling water. Cool; strain; apply as a rinse.

SAGE

Place 4 oz. sage with 2 quarts of water in an iron kettle. Let it simmer until reduced to 1 quart. Allow to stand covered for 24 hours. Strain, and apply evenly to the hair (preferably with a brush) to darken hair. Allow to dry.

HAIR GELS & SPRAYS

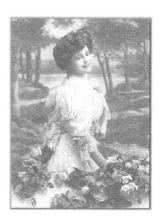

LEMON & VODKA

For a very simple hair spray, place yellow part of one lemon peel in a glass bowl and pour 1 c. boiling water over it. Let it sit several hours or overnight. Strain out peel. Stir in 1 Tb. vodka and pour into a spritzer bottle. Use on wet or dry hair. If desired, other citrus peels can be used, alone or as a combination.

PINK GRAPEFRUIT, UNFLAVORED GELATIN, GLYCERIN, & VITAMIN C

For a powerful styling gel, dissolve 1 packet gelatin in 1/2 c. warm water. Ad 1/2 c. grapefruit juice, 1 tsp. glycerin, and 1 crushed vitamin C tablet. Mix well, and refrigerate until solid (about 2 hours). To use, remove from refrigerator, allow to get to too room temperature, and give it a final thorough stirring. Use on wet or dry hair. Store in airtight container.

SUGAR

A hairspray that keeps hair in place and look thicker is made by taking 1 Tb. sugar to 1 c. warm water and mixing well. Pour into a spritzer bottle. Use before or after setting to hold style.

UNFLAVORED OR FLAVORED GELATIN

For a gel, dissolve 1 Tb. gelatin in 1 c. boiling water. Cool until firm in the refrigerator. Use on wet or dry hair to set and style it.

HAIR SHAMPOOS

ANY SHAMPOO & EGG

Mix 1 raw egg and 1 Tb. shampoo. Rinse as cool as you can stand. Adds protein.

BEER & SHAMPOO

Heat 1 c. beer in a small saucepan over medium heat and boil until the beer is reduced to 1/4 cup. Add the reduced beer to the shampoo and stir well. Adds body.

CORNMEAL

Use as a dry shampoo. Work through hair and brush through. Leaves hair clean and shiny.

EGG

Mix the white and yellow of an egg thoroughly in 1 oz. of water. Apply to hair and massage scalp vigorously with rotary motion of the hands. After the operation, rinse the hair thoroughly with clear water.

EGG YOLKS

Rub the yolks of 2 eggs into the hair, and let stand for 15-20 minutes. Shampoo with lukewarm water. Soap is not necessary, as the yolks of the eggs will lather. Use a small amount of vinegar or lemon juice in rinse water. Follow with clear water. Egg shampoo is especially useful when hair tangles easily after a permanent.

LIQUID SOAP OR INEXPENSIVE SHAMPOO, GLYCERIN, & BORAX

Mix 1 c. water, 1/2 c. liquid soap, 1/2 c. glycerin, and 1/4 c. borax powder and pour into a clean bottle. Let the mixture sit overnight to thicken.

LIQUID SOAP & LIGHT VEGETABLE OIL

Mix 1/4 c. water, 1/4 c. liquid soap, and 1/2 tsp. oil (for oily hair, omit the oil).

OLIVE OIL & LIQUID SOAP OR MILD SHAMPOO

Blend 1/2 c. water, 1/4 c. olive oil, and 1 c. soap until smooth. If hair is oily, decrease the amount of olive oil. This improves the strength of the hair.

RICE FLOUR, BAKING SODA & BORAX

For a dry shampoo, mix 1/2 c. rice flour, 1 tsp. baking soda, and 1 Tb. borax together. Massage into scalp and through hair for 15 minutes. Use a clean, dry brush to brush vigorously out all the powder. Messy, but worth it!

DORM MOM

Gukkie didn't stop at being a mother and grandmother in her own family. Oh, no.

She was a dorm mother at a woman's business college, and had influenced and inspired the lives of many women. She was so loved and respected by these women who called her, "mom."

When I was about 10 years old, I noticed the cards. Scores of them, it seemed: birthday, thank you, miss you, Christmas (and every other holiday including Mother's Day), adorned her table. She received so many of them so often that sometimes she would just bundle up the unopened ones and pack them in her suitcase when she came to visit us.

Many of those young women continued to write to Gukkie long after they had left the College.

She was Godmother to some of their children.

What secret recipe DID she have to touch these lives so deeply? When I asked her about those cards, she just giggled, blushed, and then replied, "Oh, they're just being my girls." Notice the "my" in that statement. Gukkie didn't just watch over and help guide these women---she adopted them---and they knew it. Gukkie wasn't just "doing a job." She took her position, owned it, and mastered it. How many times do we neglect to see the wonderful benefits that can spring from doing even the most tedious of jobs? The biggest benefit being the touching the life of someone else in a positive and uplifting way. That's what Gukkie would say; it wasn't the jobs she did, it was the people she came in contact with THROUGH the jobs that she took to her heart.

These days, most people just want to put in their eight hours on the job and go home. They keep to themselves and trust no one. This generation is extremely overboard in paying attention to only them. Nothing is gained by this except a momentary and temporary "fix" to fill a void of personal desire. So much more can be gained when you have the love and respect of others returned to you along the walk of growth in this life.

Essentially when you touch the life of someone else, you may not realize the extent of the impact you may have on their future. When you think about the adage, "what you put out comes back to you," you suddenly realize the scope of what positive (or, heaven forbid, negative) residue you imprint out there in the world.

Gukkie's life was so full and rich.

She lived a motto that, "a healthy, youthful, beautiful body is directly influenced by a healthy, loving spirit."

LIPS

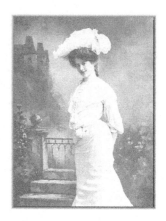

ALOE VERA GEL, COCONUT OIL & PETROLEUM JELLY

Mix 1 tsp. gel, 1/2 tsp. coconut oil and 1 tsp. jelly in small dish or cup. Gently heat the mixture until the coconut oil has melted. Pour this melted mixture into a small container. Cool completely until the mixture is solid. (15 minutes. or so).

GLYCERIN, LEMON, & CASTOR OIL

Mix 1/2 tsp. glycerin, 1/2 tsp. lemon juice, and 1/2 tsp. castor oil. Spread mixture on lips and leave on overnight. Store in refrigerator. This is said to be an overnight cure for chapped lips.

PETROLEUM JELLY & FLAVORED OIL OR EXTRACT

Take 1 Tb. of petroleum jelly and add a few drops of your favorite flavored oil or extract. Mix well in a small dish with the back of a spoon.

PETROLEUM JELLY & YOUR FAVORITE FLAVORING

Take 1 Tb. of jelly and add a few drops or 1 tsp. of your favorite flavored oil or extract (such as peppermint, coconut, cinnamon, and vanilla). Mix well in a small dish with the back of a spoon.

NAILS

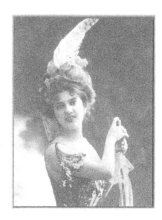

HENNA

To keep nails conditioned and strong, mix 1/2 tsp. colorless (neutral) henna and 1/2 c. boiling water. Do not use metal utensils or containers when mixing. Pour into a container with a tight-fitting lid. To use, shake solution and apply to clean, dry, nails with a cotton swab and allow to dry. Repeat 2-3 times. Do this every couple of days.

KELP

Purchased from health food and some grocery stores, dried or powdered kelp taken as a snack, salads and/or sushi helps to remedy brittle nails.

LEMON

The hands may be made white and soft and supple by daily sponging them with fresh lemon juice which further keeps the nails in good order.

OLIVE OIL

If nails are hard or brittle, immerse them in warm olive oil every night or apply small amount of Vaseline upon them.

SALT, CASTOR OIL, & WHEAT GERM OIL

To strengthen and shine nails, combine 2 tsp. salt, 2 tsp. castor oil, and 1 tsp. wheat germ oil and mix thoroughly. Pour into bottle. Shake before using. To use, rub a small amount into your nails. Leave on 3-5 minutes and tissue off. Follow up with more plain castor oil, if desired.

WITCH HAZEL, HONEY, & ALUM POWDER

For a nail hardener, combine 1 Tb. water, 1 Tb. witch hazel, 1 1/2 tsp. honey, and 1/2 tsp. alum powder. Mix well and pour into a small bottle. To use, take a cotton swab and apply the solution to clean, dry nails before buffing. Strengthens and conditions nails.

SCENTS

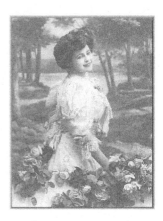

CASTOR OIL & PERFUME OR ESSENTIAL OIL

Perfect for dry skin: Mix 1/4 c. distilled water, 1/8 tsp. castor oil, and 6-8 drops of your favorite oil. Pour into a spray container and shake well.

CORNSTARCH & PERFUME OR ESSENTIAL OIL

For a scented bath powder, take 1 c. cornstarch and add 5-6 drops of perfume or oil. Mix well in a plastic bag and put into an airtight container.

FAVORITE COLOGNE

For an after-bath splash, combine 1/4 c. of cologne with 1/4 c. distilled water. Apply generously to skin.

FLOWER PETALS & VEGETABLE OIL

To make an old-fashioned Effleurage: Fill a 6-8 oz. glass jar with 1-2 c. flower petals (rose, lavender, lilac, and gardenia), and cover them with 1 c. light vegetable oil (all the oil may not be used). Place jar in sunny spot. Let sit for 24 hours. Strain off oil and discard petals. Add fresh petals for 3-4 days until you have the desired scent. To keep the scent from changing, use 1 or 2 drops of glycerin or castor oil. Store in a cool place in an air-tight container. If an alcohol base is desired, mix the solution with an equal amount of vodka and let stand for a day, then shake. Do this every day for a week. The vodka will absorb the scent from the oil.

PEPPERMINT OIL, VODKA, & CORNSTARCH

A refreshing powder for hot, sticky days: Mix 1/2 tsp. peppermint oil and 1 tsp. vodka. Place cornstarch in a plastic bag and add the peppermint mixture. Seal bag and mix well. Put into an airtight container.

VODKA & PERFUME OR ESSENTIAL OIL

For a wonderful daytime cologne and make your perfume or oil go an extra mile, mix 1/4 c. vodka, 1/4 c. water, and 2-3 drops of your favorite oil. To use, spray or splash the cologne onto the skin or hair. (I love this one...it works so well, you could bottle and sell it).

SLENDERIZERS

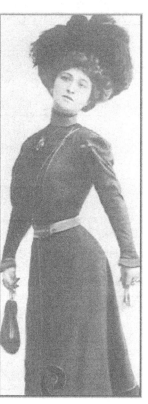

ACUPRESSURE

The next time you feel hungry; squeeze your earlobes for 1 minute.

CABBAGE

Substitute a cabbage salad with lemon dressing for a meal. You can also boil cabbage and drink the juice throughout the day. EXCELLENT treatment for obesity.

CHINESE GREEN TEA

Effective at getting rid of fat, drink up to 3 cups of green tea daily. Regular tea can also be used with a lesser effect.

FENNEL

"Take fennel and seethe it in water, a very good quantity, and wring out the juice thereof when it is sod, and drink it first and last (presumably on getting up in the morning and before retiring at night), and it shall swage him or her."

HERBAL BODY WRAP USING 1 C. OF YOUR FAVORITE HERBS

Take 1 cup of your favorite herb(s) such as chamomile, rosemary, sage, lavender, and pour them into a large sinkful or bucketful of very hot (but not boiling) water. Allow to steep for 5 minutes. Into this place a large beach towel or cotton sheet. Lay a plastic tarp or drop cloth on your bed. Wring out the towel/sheets and wrap them around your body. Have someone cover you the rest of the way with the plastic. Cover over this with blankets and rest for 10 minutes. (Don't go to sleep, here. 10 minutes. is sufficient). Unwrap and do not shower for 24 hours, although you can wash your hair in the sink. (The herbal properties continue to work during this time). This is said to be slimming, but if nothing else, it makes you feel terrific.

KELP

Purchased from health food stores, dried or powdered kelp taken daily helps to step up metabolism. Kelp also acts as a natural diuretic to get rid of excess water weight and bloating associated with menstruation.

LIME JUICE & HONEY

Mix 1 tsp. fresh honey with the juice of a half of lime in a glass of lukewarm water. Fast with this drink, drinking it at regular intervals.

SASSAFRAS

An 80-year old recipe book says: " A strong decoction of Sassafras, (obtained at herb shops), drunk frequently, will reduce the flesh as rapidly as any remedy known. A strong infusion is made at the rate of 1 oz. of Sassafras to a quart of water. Boil it 1/2 hour very slowly and let it stand till cold, heating again, if desired. Keep it from the air."

TOMATO

Eat one or two ripe tomatoes early in the morning as breakfast for a couple of months. This works especially well for obesity and tomatoes provide valuable nutrients during weight loss.

SOAPS, CLEANSERS, & SCRUBS

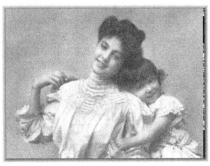

ALOE VERA GEL & WHOLE MILK

Mix 1/4 c. aloe vera gel and 2 Tb. whole milk. Store in refrigerator. Cleanse face with mixture. Rinse with tepid water.

AVOCADO OR BANANA, EGG & MILK

For a cleanser, blend a half-ripened banana or avocado with a beaten egg yolk and 1/2 c. milk and apply gently to the face. Leave on for 5 minutes. Rinse.

CORNSTARCH & GLYCERIN

Mix 2 Tb. cornstarch, 2 Tb. glycerin, and 1/2 c. water until smooth. Heat in a small pan placed in a water bath inside another pan. Heat until thick and clear; it will have the consistency of pudding. Do not boil. Cool completely, Use in place of soap to cleanse your skin. (If jelly is too thick, you may thin it by adding a little water, one Tb. at a time, until you reach the desired consistency.)

GRAPEFRUIT, OLIVE OIL & BORAX

Mix the peel from one grapefruit, 1/2 c. olive oil, 2 Tb. grapefruit juice, and 1/2 tsp. borax powder in a ceramic bowl. Heat for 2 minutes until very hot but not boiling. Cool. Pour the mixture through a strainer to remove all grapefruit peel. Store in airtight container. Use to cleanse face. Good for oily skin.

LIQUID SOAP, GLYCERIN, & OLIVE OIL

Mix 1 tsp. soap, 2 Tb. water, 2 Tb. glycerin, and 1/2 c. olive oil in a blender or by hand until smooth and creamy. Massage into skin to cleanse.

LIQUID SOAP & HONEY

Stir together 2 Tb. soap, 1/4 c. honey, and 1/4 c. distilled water. Mix well but do not beat. Pour a small amount in your hand and massage gently into your skin or hair. Rinse thoroughly with tepid water.

OATMEAL, CORNMEAL & WHEAT GERM

Combine 2 Tbs. of each and store in an airtight container. To use, combine a tsp. or two with equal parts of water or cleanser to create a paste. Massage into skin and rinse.

OLIVE OIL & LYE GRANULES

This recipe is said to make the best basic Castile Soap: Heat 2 c. olive oil to about 85 degrees. Dissolve 1/2 c. lye granules in 2 c. cold water and cool to 70 degrees. Pour the lye mixture into the oil, pouring a slowly in a thin, steady stream with slow, even stirring. No heat should be on during this time. Continue stirring until a thick, honey-like texture is obtained - which should take about 15-20 minutes. If the soap mixture does not become thick within 30 minutes and there's a greasy layer on top, it may be too warm. Set it in cool water and keep stirring from the sides and bottom. However, if it's lumpy, it may be too cold. Set it in a pan of warm water and stir until lumps disappear.

PLAIN YOGURT, LIGHT OIL, & LEMON

Mix together 1/2 c. yogurt, 1 Tb. oil, and 1 1/2 tsp. fresh lemon juice. Store in the refrigerator and use to cleanse your face. Rinse well with tepid water and pat dry.

SUGAR & LEMON

While washing your face with soap or other cleanser, add a tsp. of sugar to the lather and rotate on your face in a circular motion. Rinse with a mixture of equal parts of lemon juice and water. Rinse with clear water.

SUPER SIMPLE OATMEAL SOAP

Place 1 c. grated (1 3-oz. bar) castile soap in a double-broiler or ceramic bowl in a pan of water on the stove. Pour 1/4 c. water over the soap and stir over medium heat to dissolve all the soap in the water. When the soap is dissolved, add 2 Tbs. oatmeal and stir well. Pour into a greased mold (use petroleum jelly or vegetable shortening). Let cool and gently remove soap from mold. Let sit a few days before using (to dry it out.)

GUKKIE'S ANTI-WRINKLE FORMULA

Some people never seem to age. Gukkie was one of those lucky (or is *blessed?*) ones.

She was very petite, fun and I will always remember her face being soft and smelling wonderful when I kissed her. Gukkie didn't wear many cosmetics. Maybe lipstick---only when she got dressed up.

When I grew later in years, I asked her for her secret. Was I surprised to find that her secret could not be bought! No special formula there!

Her answer to my inquiry was so simple, I just didn't "get it" at first. Now at the age of 50, I do.

I must backtrack to an incident which illustrates Gukkie's anti-wrinkle "formula" perfectly.

One Christmas, my paternal great-grandmother and Gukkie, my maternal great-grandmother, sat on a "divan" and started to giggle. No one knew why. It must have been their own special "moment" or something.

Anyway, my dad caught this exchange on film. These two older women in the photograph are trying their hardest not to be obnoxious. Gukkie with her one hand over her mouth, and my other great-grandmother smiling as if to suppress a moth ready to burst from her mouth if she opened it.

Gukkie's formula for countering the aging process:

1. Smile. Life is *not* all *that* serious. Take advantage of moments to laugh.

2. When you boil potatoes, hold your face over the steam. You do not need to cover your head (unless someone comes to your door and your hair is completely matted to your scalp).

3. Use Ivory soap.

Gukkie was always the first one to giggle over SOMETHING. She always found something to snicker over during the course of the days' activities and sometimes, trials. She would, at the very least, find something ironic about how God sometimes uses humor to wake us up and smell the coffee---and how He shows us the many times how silly we can sometimes be and think.

Also, laughter aids digestion after a heavy meal. Laughter puts life's trials into perspective.

WRINKLES

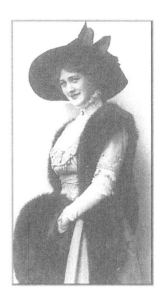

CUCUMBER JUICE & EGG WHITE

Use the white of one egg beaten stiff, blended with 4 Tbs. cucumber juice. Give the mask about 15 minutes. to dry before rinsing off. Tightens the skin and temporarily removes unsightly pouches and wrinkles.

MAYONNAISE

Apply and let sit for 15-30 minutes. Safflower oil, lanolin, and vitamins A, D, and E oils are also used with good results.

POTATO

Oh my, Gukkie and her potatoes...but boy, did she look great through the years. Guess we won't poo-poo this one: Place slices of raw potatoes on the eyelids to reduce wrinkling and puffiness.

WATERMELON

Take a good-size piece (with plenty of the red part attached) watermelon and rub the face, neck, and arm briskly until the pulp of the melon has worked off almost to the rind. It is said to remove or moderate wrinkles. (The massaging effect probably is also important for results.)

HEALTH SECTION

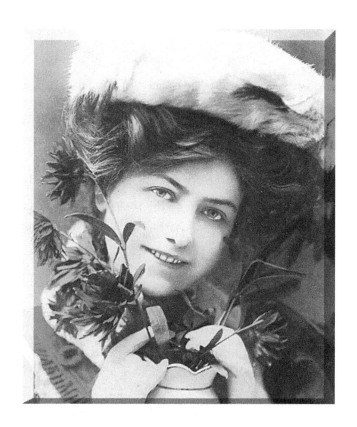

ACHES & PAINS

BUTTERMILK

A common treatment for sore muscles and cramps involves hot compresses soaked in buttermilk.

CHAMOMILE & OLIVE OIL

For an oil rub for muscle cramps, fill a glass jar with chamomile flowers and add enough olive oil to fill the jar. Screw down the cap tightly and leave in the sun for 3 weeks, adding more olive oil and flowers as the mixture settles. Strain off the oil, pressing the flowers to extract the last drop.

FISH

A daily serving of fresh fish or fish oil capsules helps to give relief of arthritis and other aches and pains.

GARLIC

Take 2-3 cloves every morning will help get rid of back pain. Garlic oil that is spread on the back is especially effective: fry 10 garlic cloves in about ¼ c. oil. After the oil cools, rub vigorously on the back then allow to remain there for three hours. Then take a warm-water bath.

LEMON

Mix a bit of salt to the juice of one lemon and take twice daily to treat back pain.

LIGHT VEGETABLE OIL & CAMPHOR OIL

Mix 1/2 c. of both oils together and pour into a bottle. This is used in a massage for sore muscles.

ONIONS & HONEY

Smear a mixture of chopped onions and honey on the area to soothe muscle aches.

OLIVE OIL & CAMPHOR

Take equal parts of olive oil and camphor and apply red peppers externally for muscle aches.

POTATO

Grate enough raw potato to make a poultice and apply to the affected area for back pain.

RED PEPPER & VEGETABLE OIL

For external application to help treat pain, mix 1/4 to 1/2 tsp. hot red pepper per cup of warm vegetable oil and rub it into the affected area.

VINEGAR

Vinegar compresses are very good for relieving muscle aches. Additionally, use a cup at a time in the bath to alleviate muscle soreness. Splash it on directly on shoulders, arms, chest, and torso to restore flagging energy.

ALCOHOLISM

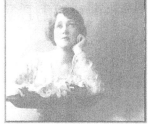

APPLES

Apples are another effective remedy for alcoholism. A generous intake of apples helps remove intoxication and reduces the craving for wines and other intoxicating liquors.

BITTER GOURD

The juice of the leaves of bitter gourd is an antidote for alcohol intoxication. It is also useful for a liver damaged due to alcoholism. Three teaspoons of this juice, mixed with a glass of butter milk, should be taken every morning for a month.

CELERY

The juice of raw celery has also been found useful in alcoholism. It exercises a sobering effect on the patient and is an antidote to alcohol. Half a glass of celery juice mixed with an equal quantity of water should be taken once daily for a month.

DATES

Dates are considered beneficial in the treatment of alcoholism. The patient should drink half a glass of water in which four or five dates have been rubbed together. This remedy should be taken twice daily for a month. It will bring definite relief.

GRAPES

The most important home remedy for alcoholism is an exclusive diet, for a month or so, of grapes. Since this fruit contains the purest form of alcohol, it is an ideal yet healthy substitute for alcohol. Alcoholics should take three meals a day of fresh grapes at five-hourly intervals. The success of this treatment also depends on the determination of the alcoholic to stop drinking.

ALLERGIES & HAY FEVER

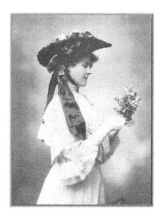

BANANAS

One or two bananas a day are useful for skin rashes, digestive disorders, or asthma. The fruit does, however; cause allergic reactions in certain sensitive persons, and they should avoid it

BLACKSTRAP MOLASSES

Take 1 Tb. before or at the onset of an attack daily.

FENUGREEK SEED

Steep 1 tsp. steep in 1 c. water, covered, for 10 minutes. Drink 1 c. a day to help hay fever symptoms.

HONEY

Eat teaspoons of honey to avoid an attack or relieve one. Bee pollen, in same amounts, also offers relief. It is best to use honey or pollen from your area.

HONEYCOMB

Take one chew of honeycomb every hour for 4-6 hours to relieve sinus attacks.

HORSERADISH

A spoonful of Japanese wasabe or horseradish makes your eyes water and clears your sinuses. A daily dosage is necessary only until the symptoms of your allergy subside. Thereafter, you need only a few tsp. of horseradish each month to prevent another allergy attack.

LIME

Lime is considered an effective remedy for any kind of allergy. Half a lime may be squeezed in a glass of lukewarm water and sweetened with a teaspoon of honey. It can be taken once daily first thing in the morning for several months. This remedy not only flushes the system of toxins but also acts as an anti toxic and anti allergic agent. However, those who are allergic to citrus fruits should not take recourse to this remedy.

SALT

You may greatly relieve the irritation in the nose at once by sniffing salt water up the nose. For this purpose, dissolve one heaping tsp. of salt in a pint of warm water. Gargle with this solution, and blow the nose clearly of mucous before sniffing up the nose.

VEGETABLE JUICES

A quantity of 500 ml carrot juice or a combination of carrot juice with beet and cucumber juices, has been found beneficial in the treatment of allergies. In the case of mixed juices, 100 ml each of beet and cucumber juices should be mixed with 300 mi of carrot juice to prepare 500 ml or half a liter of mixed juice. This should be taken once daily.

VITAMINS

Certain nutrients have been found beneficial in the prevention and treatment of allergies. Often the intake of vitamin B5 or pantothenic acid brings exceptional relief to the sufferer. This vitamin may be taken in a dose of 100 mg daily for a month. In such cases, liberal amounts of pantothenic acid helps even though the recovery takes several weeks. A dose of 400 mg of vitamin E taken daily for four to six weeks is also beneficial as this vitamin possesses effective anti-allergic properties.

ANEMIA

ALMONDS

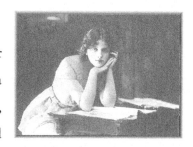

Almonds contain copper to the extent of 1.15 mg per 100 gm. The copper along with iron and vitamins acts as a catalyst in the synthesis of hemoglobin. Almonds are, therefore; a useful remedy for anemia. Seven almonds should be soaked in water for about two hours and ground into a paste after removing the thin red skin. This paste may be eaten once daily in the morning for three months.

BEE POLLEN

Bee pollen is a biological stimulant that increases the red blood cells in bone marrow. You should take 1 teaspoon of bee pollen daily to treat anemia.

BEETS

Beets are very helpful in curing anemia. Beet juice contains potassium, phosphorus, calcium, sulphur, iodine, iron, copper, carbohydrates, protein, fat, vitamins B1, B2, B6, niacin, and vitamin P. With their high iron content, beets help in the formation of red blood cells. The juice of red heel strengthens the body's powers of resistance and has proved to be an excellent remedy for anemia, especially for children and teenagers, where oilier blood-fanning remedies have failed.

BRANDY

Add 2 Tbs. of ground orange peel, ½ tsp. of ground ginger, and 2 Tbs. of chamomile to 2 c. of boiling water. Steep until cool. Strain, and add to 1 c. of brandy. Dosage is ½ c. in the morning and again in the evening. Said to be a blood builder.

COMFREY

Put 1 tsp each of dried comfrey, fenugreek seed, and dandelion in 2 c. of boiling water. Steep 10 minutes. Strain and add honey as a sweetener. Drink after meals. Said to be a blood builder.

FENUGREEK

The leaves of fenugreek help in blood formation. The cooked leaves should be taken by adolescent girls to prevent anemia, which may occur due to the onset of puberty and menstruation. The seeds of fenugreek are also a valuable cure for anemia, being rich in iron.

HONEY

Honey is remarkable for building hemoglobin in the body. This is largely due to the iron, copper, and manganese contained in it.

IRON BOOSTER RECIPE

Leaves of 3 beetroots

3-5 carrots

½ green pepper

½ apple, seeded

Extract the juice from each and mix well.

LETTUCE

Lettuce is another effective remedy for this ailment, as it contains a considerable amount of iron. It can, therefore; be used as a good tonic food for anemia. The iron in it is easily absorbed by the body.

SESAME SEEDS

Black sesame seeds, as a rich source of iron, are valuable in anemia. After soaking one teaspoon of the seeds in warm water for a couple of hours, they seeds should be ground and strained, and then mixed with a cup of milk and sweetened with sugar. This emulsion should be given to patients suffering from anemia.

SOY BEANS

Soy beans are rich in iron and also have a high protein value. As most anemic patients usually also suffer from a weak digestion, it should be given to them in a very light form, preferably in the form of milk, which can be easily digested.

SPINACH

This leafy vegetable is a valuable source of high grade iron. After its absorption, it helps in the formation of hemoglobin and red blood cells. It is thus beneficial in building up the blood, and in the prevention and treatment of anemia.

VINEGAR & MOLASSES

Mix 2 teaspoons each of apple cider vinegar and blackstrap molasses with water or tea to strengthen the blood.

VITAMIN B-12

Vitamin B12 is needed for preventing or curing anemia. This vitamin is usually found in animal protein, especially in meats such as kidney and liver. There are, however; other equally good sources of vitamin B12 such as dairy products that also contain some B12.

ANOREXIA

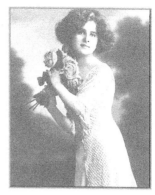

APPLES

Apples are another variety of fruit useful in anorexia. They help digestion by stimulating the flow of pepsin, a protein-digesting enzyme, in the stomach.

GARLIC

Garlic possesses a special property to stimulate the digestive tone of the system and improve appetite. A soup prepared from this vegetable can be of immense help to a patient suffering from anorexia. Three or four cloves of raw garlic should be boiled in a cup of water. This soup can be reinforced with the juice of half a lemon and taken twice daily,

GINGER

The use of ginger is valuable in the loss of appetite. About five grams of this vegetable should be ground and licked with a little salt once a day for the treatment of this condition.

LIME

Lime is also a valuable remedy for restoring a lost appetite. A preparation made from this fruit and ginger has been found very effective in overcoming this condition. About one teaspoon of the juice of lime should be mixed with an equal quantity of the juice of ginger. One gram of rock salt should be added to this mixture. It should then be placed in sunlight for three days. A teaspoon taken after each meal will tone up the digestive system and improve the appetite.

ORANGES

Oranges are an extremely useful remedy for anorexia. They stimulate the flow of digestive juices, thereby improving digestion and increasing appetite. One or two oranges a day are advised.

SOUR GRAPES

Sour grapes are another effective remedy for anorexia.

ARTERIOSCLEROSIS

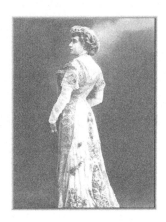

GARLIC & ONIONS

Include raw or cooked in the daily diet to prevent the development of arteriosclerosis.

HONEY

Add to 1 glass of water 1 tsp. of honey and some lemon juice. Drink before bedtime.

LEMON PEEL

Cut up the peel of one or two lemons finely. Cover with warm water and allow to stand for about 12 hours. Take 1 tsp. every three hours or immediately before or after a meal. One of the most effective treatments.

PARSLEY

Simmer 1 tsp. of dry parsley in 1 c. water for a few minutes. This tea can be taken 2-3 times daily.

VEGETABLE JUICES

Beet, carrot, and spinach juices, taken daily, help to treat arteriosclerosis.

ARTHRITIS

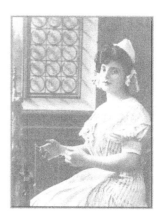

ALFALFA

A tea made bum the herb alfalfa, especially from its seeds, has shown beneficial results in the treatment of arthritis. One teaspoon of alfalfa seeds may be added to one cup of water. Three to four cups of this tea should be taken daily by arthritics for at least two weeks.

APPLE CIDER VINEGAR

Mix 4 cups of apple cider vinegar to 4 cups of hot water. Dip a cloth into the hot vinegar water and apply as a compress to the affected area. Put a heating pad over the compress and keep on for 30 minutes.

ARTHRITIS COCKTAIL

2 Tbs. honey

1 ½ c. water

1 oz. apple cider vinegar

Drink once daily to rid symptoms in about a month.

BANANAS

Bananas, being a rich source of vitamin B6, have proved useful in the treatment of arthritis. A diet of only bananas for three or four days is advised in treating this condition. The patient may eat eight or nine bananas daily during this period and nothing else.

BARLEY TEA

Barley tea is an excellent way to treat arthritis. Make a tea by soaking 1 cup of unhulled barley in 8 cups of boiling water for 3 hours. Strain and keep refrigerated. Drink 1 cup twice daily.

BREWER'S YEAST

Put two tablespoons of Brewer's yeast in a glass of milk or juice and drink every morning.

CALCIUM

Studies have shown that calcium can help arthritis. Several patients have discovered that joint pains have either been relieved or have disappeared entirely after taking calcium. This mineral should be taken in the form of calcium lactate. Two teaspoons of calcium lactate, each teaspoon providing 400 mg of Absorbable calcium, may be taken three times daily in water, before meals for at least four months.

COCONUT OR MUSTARD OIL

Warm coconut oil or mustard oil, mixed with two or three pieces of camphor should be massaged on stiff and aching joints. It will increase blood supply, and reduce inflammation and stiffness with the gentle warmth produced while massaging.

COD LIVER OIL

Put 2 tablespoons of cod-liver oil in a glass of warm milk and drink twice daily. This will reduce inflammation of the joint tissue, thus reducing pain.

COPPER

Drinking water kept overnight in a copper container accumulates traces of copper, which is said to strengthen the muscular system. A copper ring or bracelet is worn for the same reason.

GARLIC

Garlic is another effective remedy for arthritis. It contains an anti-inflammatory property which accounts for its effectiveness in the treatment of this disease. Garlic may be taken raw or cooked according to individual preference.

HERBS

Mix 1 tablespoon each of corn silk, broom flowers, skullcap, and boneset. Pour 1 cup boiling water over 1 tablespoon of herb mixture and steep 15 minutes. Strain and sweeten. Drink with meals.

LIME

Lime has also been found beneficial as a home remedy for arthritis. The citric acid found in lime is a solvent of uric acid, which is the primary cause of some types of arthritis. The juice of one lime, diluted with water, may be taken once a day, preferably first thing in the morning.

OTHER RAW JUICES

One cup of green juice, extracted from any green leafy vegetable, mixed in equal proportions with carrot, celery, and red beet juices is good for arthritis. The alkaline action of raw juices dissolves the accumulation of deposits around the joints and in other tissues. A cup of fresh pineapple juice is also valuable, as the enzyme bromelain in fresh pineapple juice reduces swelling and inflammation in osteoarthritis and rheumatoid arthritis.

PARSLEY

Add 1 teaspoon of fresh parsley to 1 cup of boiling water. Let steep 15 minutes. Strain and sweeten. Add 1/2 teaspoon of fresh ginger to the tea and drink hot. Drink at every meal.

POTATO JUICE

The raw potato juice therapy is considered one of the most successful biological treatments for rheumatic and arthritic conditions. It has been used in folk medicine for centuries. The traditional method of preparing potato juice is to cut a medium-sized potato into thin slices, without peeling the skin, and place the slices overnight in a large glass filled with cold water. The water should be drunk in the morning on an empty stomach. Fresh juice can also be extracted from potatoes. A medium-sized potato should be diluted with a cup of water and drunk first thing in the morning.

RAW JUICES

One cup of green juice, extracted from any green leafy vegetable, mixed in equal proportions with carrot, celery, and red beet juices is good for arthritis. The alkaline action of raw juices dissolves the accumulation of deposits around the joints and in other tissues. A cup of fresh pineapple juice is also valuable, as the enzyme bromelain in fresh pineapple juice reduces swelling and inflammation in osteoarthritis and rheumatoid arthritis.

SESAME SEEDS

A teaspoon of black sesame seeds, soaked in a quarter cup of water and kept overnight, has been found to be effective in preventing frequent joint pains. The water in which the seeds are soaked should also be taken along with the seeds first thing in the morning.

ASTHMA

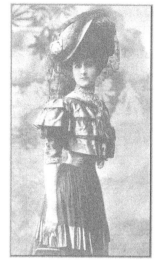

ALOE VERA

If you suffer from asthma, boil some aloe vera leaves in a pan of water and inhale the vapors. Put a towel over the head and pan to get the full effects of the vapors.

COLTSFOOT

Add 1 tablespoon each of coltsfoot, mullein, thyme, and lobelia to 2 cups of water. Simmer at least half hour, covered. Strain and add 2 cups of honey. Take by the tablespoon until relief is obtained. Flavoring, such as oil of peppermint, may be added if desired.

COPPER

One of the preventive measures to stop attacks of asthma is to drink water which has been kept overnight in a copper vessel. This water, with traces of copper in it, is believed to change one's constitutional tendency to get respiratory problems.

CRANBERRY JUICE

Cranberry juice is very good for treating asthma attacks, as it contains an ingredient that dilates the bronchial tubes. Cook and mash cranberries. Place in a tightly closed glass container and refrigerate. When needed during an attack, add 3 teaspoons of the mashed cranberries to a cup of hot water. Sip while the water is hot.

FIGS

Among fruits, figs have, proved very valuable in asthma. They give comfort to the patient by draining off the phlegm. Three or four dry figs should he cleaned thoroughly with warm water and soaked overnight They should be taken first thing in the morning, along with the water in which they were soaked.

GARLIC

Garlic is another effective home remedy for asthma. 10 garlic cloves, boiled in 30 ml of milk, make an excellent medicine for the early stages of asthma. This mixture should be taken once daily by the patient. Steaming ginger tea with two minced garlic cloves in it, can also help to keep the problem under control, and should be taken in the morning and evening.

GINGER

A teaspoon of fresh ginger juice, mixed with a cup of fenugreek decoction and honey to taste, acts as an excellent expectorant m cases of asthma. The decoction of fenugreek can be made by mixing one tablespoon of fenugreek seeds in a cupful of water. This remedy should be taken once in the morning and once in the evening.

HONEY

Honey is one of the most common home remedies for asthma. It is said that if a jug of honey is held under the nose of ail asthma patient, and he inhales the air that comes into contact with it, he starts breathing easier and deeper. The effect lasts for an hour or so. One to two teaspoons of honey provide relief. Honey can also be taken in a cup of milk or water. Honey thins out accumulated mucus and helps its elimination from the respiratory passages. It also tones up the pulmonary lining and thereby prevents the production of mucus in future. Some authorities recommend one-year old honey for asthma and respiratory diseases.

HONEYSUCKLE TEA

Many people drink honeysuckle tea to help with chronic asthma. Put 1 tablespoon of the grated root of honeysuckle in 1 cup of water. Boil gently for 10 minutes. Strain and sweeten. Drink daily.

HORSERADISH

Add several tablespoons of freshly grated horseradish to 1 cup of milk. Simmer for 10 minutes and strain. Drink as necessary to obtain relief.

IRISH MOSS

Mix 1 tablespoon each of boneset, Irish moss, coltsfoot, mullein, thyme, rosemary, valerian, and lobelia. Add 1 teaspoon of the herbal mixture to 1 cup of boiling water. Cover and steep for 15 minutes. Strain. Peppermint or cherry oil may be added for flavoring if desired. Drink 4 cups daily to obtain relief.

LEMON

Lemon is another fruit found beneficial in the treatment of asthma. The juice of one lemon, dilated in a glass of water and taken with meals will bring good results.

MULLEIN ROOT

Clean the root of mullein very carefully. Add 1 cup of the chopped root to 2 cups of water. Bring to a boil and simmer until the liquid is reduced by half. Strain well and add 1 cup of honey. Give 2 tablespoons as needed. This is also good to use during colds, as it helps to remove phlegm.

ONIONS

Make fresh daily. Cut an onion into very thin slices and place in a bowl. Cover onion slices with honey and let sit overnight. The next day, scrape the honey from the onion slices and take 1 teaspoon 3-4 times daily.

POTATO

Boil several potatoes. Place in a basin and cover the head and basin with a towel to get the most from the steam.

SUNFLOWER OR CORN OIL

Take 1 Tb. before bed to help you breathe easier through the night.

TUMERIC

Turmeric is also regarded as an effective remedy for bronchial asthma. The patient should be given a teaspoon of turmeric powder with a glass of milk two or three times daily. It acts best when taken on an empty stomach.

BLADDER INFECTION

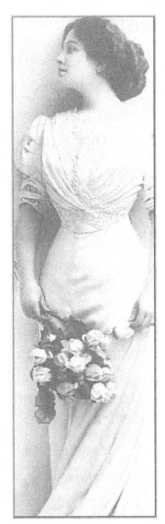

(CYSTITIS)

BARLEY

Half a glass each of barley gruel, mixed with buttermilk and the juice of half a lime, is an excellent diuretic. It is beneficial in the treatment of cystitis, and may be taken twice daily.

BLADDER CLEANSING TEA

3 teaspoons marshmallow root

2 teaspoons dandelion leaf

2 teaspoons crushed juniper berries

3 teaspoons nettle

4 cups water

Simmer marshmallow root in water in a covered pot for 5 minutes. Remove from heat and add dandelion leaf, juniper berries, and nettle. Cover, and steep for 15 minutes. Strain and drink 3-4 cups throughout the day.

CUCUMBER JUICE

Cucumber juice is one of the most useful home remedies in the treatment of cystitis. It is a very effective diuretic. A cup of this juice, mixed with one teaspoon of honey and a tablespoon of fresh lime juice, should be given three times daily.

GOLDENSEAL

Goldenseal has anti-inflammatory and astringent properties that help to soothe inflamed mucous membranes. As with uva ursi, the natural antibiotic in goldenseal is most effective in an alkaline environment, so avoid eating acidifying foods while you are taking the herb. Pour one cup of boiling water over one teaspoon of powdered herb. Steep 10 minutes, strain, and drink three cups a day. Goldenseal is extremely bitter and is easiest to take as a liquid extract or in capsules. Take one-half to one teaspoon of extract or two to three capsules three times a day. Because it is a uterine stimulant, goldenseal should not be used during pregnancy.

INFECTION-FIGHTING MIXTURE

1 ounce uva ursi extract

1/2 ounce goldenseal extract

1/2 Ounce echinacea root extract

Combine extracts in a dark glass bottle and shake well. Take 1 teaspoon four times a day in a small amount of warm water.

JUNIPER

Juniper berries contain an aromatic oil that has antimicrobial and diuretic properties. It steps up the fluid filtering rate of the kidneys, which increases urine output. Juniper has a sweet, pungent, and astringent flavor. To make a tea, pour one cup of boiling water over one teaspoon of crushed berries, cover, and steep for 20 minutes. Strain, and drink up to three cups a day. Overuse of juniper can irritate the kidneys, and the herb should not be used for more than four to six weeks at a time. If you have kidney disease or are pregnant, do not use juniper.

LEMON

Lemon has proved valuable in cystitis. A teaspoon of lemon juice should be put in 180 ml of boiling water. It should then be allowed to cool and 60 ml of this water should be taken every two hours from 8 a.m. to noon for the treatment of this condition. This eases the burning sensation and also stops bleeding in cystitis.

MARSHMALLOW

While it won't fight infection as do uva ursi or goldenseal, it makes a soothing tea that helps to cleanse the bladder. Marshmallow has a pleasant, sweet flavor. Simmer one teaspoon of chopped dried root in one cup of boiling water in a covered pot for five minutes. Remove from heat and steep an additional 10 minutes. Strain, and drink three to four cups throughout the day.

SANDALWOOD OIL

The oil of sandalwood is also considered valuable in this disease. This oil should be given in doses of five drops in the beginning and gradually increased to 10 to 30 drops.

SPINACH

A quantity of 100 ml of fresh spinach juice, taken with an equal quantity of tender coconut water twice a day, is considered beneficial in the treatment of cystitis. It acts as a very effective and safe diuretic due to the combined action of both nitrates and potassium.

UVA URSI

The antibacterial component of Uva Ursi seems to be most effective in an alkaline environment, so it may be helpful while using the herb to avoid cranberry juice, citrus, tomatoes, and other foods that might acidify the urine. Uva Ursi has an astringent but not unpleasant flavor. Make a tea by pouring one cup of boiling water over two teaspoons of dried leaves. Steep for 10 minutes, strain, and drink three cups a day. As an alternative, take one-half teaspoon of liquid extract or two capsules three times a day. Although Uva Ursi is safe when used in recommended amounts, don't exceed the recommended dosage or use it for more than two weeks, because in high doses it can cause nausea and irritate the kidneys. Do not take uva ursi during pregnancy.

Aroma Therapy for Cyctitis

Aromatherapy essential oils can be added to baths, compresses, and massage oils to help to relieve urinary tract infections. Sitz baths can ease the pelvic pain that sometimes accompanies an infection. Add five drops each of juniper and sandalwood essential oils to the tub.

JUNIPER A potent detoxifying oil with diuretic properties and is specifically an antiseptic for the urinary tract. It has a pungent, sweet, woodsy fragrance. Do not use juniper during pregnancy.

SANDALWOOD

An antiseptic and diuretic and is used extensively in alternative medicine for treating urinary tract infections. It has a complex, rich, woodsy and sweet scent.

TEA TREE OIL

A potent antiseptic that directly kills the bacteria that cause urinary tract infections. If you suffer frequently from this infection, add two drops of tea tree oil to one cup of warm water and use regularly as a genital wash after bowel movements and following intercourse. Tea tree oil has a pungent, camphor-like scent.

AROMATHERAPY BATH

2 cups Epsom salts

1 cup baking soda

6 drops sandalwood essential oil

4 drops juniper essential oil

Fill bathtub with comfortably hot water, adding Epsom salts and baking soda while the tub is filling. Add sandalwood and juniper essential oils just before entering the tub. Soak for 15 to 20 minutes.

MASSAGE OIL

1 ounce almond oil

7 drops sandalwood essential oil

5 drops juniper essential oil

1/4 teaspoon vitamin E oil

Combine oils and store in a dark glass bottle. Use as a massage oil over the abdomen and lower back.

BOILS

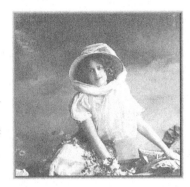

BACON

To bring a boil to a head, place a small piece of fatty bacon over the boil and bandage it. Leave on overnight. The head should be ready to remove by the next morning.

BITTER GOURD

Bitter gourd is another effective home remedy for blood-filled boils. A cupful of fresh juice of this vegetable, mixed with a teaspoon of lime juice, should be taken, sip by sip, on an empty stomach daily for a few months to treat this condition.

CREAM

Milk cream is beneficial in the treatment of boils. One teaspoon of milk cream, mixed with half a teaspoon of vinegar, and a pinch of turmeric powder, makes an excellent poultice. It helps in ripening the blood boils and in their healing without allowing them to become septic.

CUMIN SEEDS

Cumin seeds are beneficial in the treatment of boils. The seeds should be ground in water and made into a paste. This paste can be applied to boils with beneficial results.

GARLIC AND ONION

Garlic and onions have proved most effective among the several home remedies found beneficial in the treatment of boils. The juice of garlic or onion may be applied externally on boils to help ripen them, break them, and evacuate the pus. An equal quantity of the juices of these two vegetables can also be applied with beneficial results. Eating of two to three pods of garlic during meals will also bring good results.

LEMON JUICE

Soak a piece of bread in lemon juice and apply to the boil. Cover with a loose bandage and try to leave on overnight.

LINSEED OIL

Apply linseed oil to the boil to soften and aid in healing.

PANSY

Native Americans used wild heartsease (pansy) to draw boils. It was ground up and placed on the boil, bandaged and left on overnight.

PARSLEY

Take a handful of crushed parsley and wrap in cheesecloth. Apply to the boil and wrap a hot cloth around the area. Repeat, covering the area with the hot cloth for about 15 minutes.

TURMERIC

Application of turmeric powder on boils speeds up the healing process. In the case of fresh boils, a few dry roots of turmeric are roasted, the ashes dissolved in a cupful of water, and then applied over the affected portion. This solution enables the boils to ripen and burst.

BRONCHITIS & ASTHMA

ALMOND

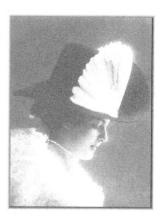

An emulsion of almonds is useful in bronchial diseases, including bronchitis. It is prepared by making a powder of seven kernels of almonds and mixing the powdered kernels in a cup of orange or lemon juice. This emulsion may be taken once daily at night.

APPLES & HONEY

For bronchitis and severe coughs, bake an apple with honey and serve mashed with butter (another Gukkie favorite). Daily drinking of apple juice also helps prevent upper respiratory ailments.

ASPARAGUS

Pour 1 can of asparagus in the blender. Liquefy and refrigerate. Drink 1/4 cup every morning and before retiring to bed. Add water to make a hot drink if desired. You should notice quite an improvement in chronic bronchitis in a few weeks.

BEE POLLEN

Allergy related bronchitis is best treated with bee pollen. One teaspoon of pollen granules should be taken daily. During an attack, vitamin C should be taken in doses of 1000 mg every hour. Vitamin C has an anti-infection action and will help the immune system to regain balance, enabling it to fight the infection.

CHICKEN SOUP

Cook chicken with water, celery, onions, carrots, and a garlic clove or two, until the chicken falls off the bone. Strain the broth, discarding any fat. Put thin slices of lemon on top and serve the broth. Vitamin C, onion, and garlic are the big fighters.

CHILI PEPPERS

For bronchitis, eat a hot chili pepper. The eyes water and the nose runs. Lungs and bronchial passages also produce watery secretions. The mucus in the lungs is thinned and coughing is eased. Ease a fiery mouth afterward by eating some cool yogurt or bread, or drink some milk.

COFFEE

Drink two 8-oz. cups of strong brewed coffee for asthma.

COMFREY

Put 1/4 ounce of comfrey leaves in 2 cups of boiling water. Cover and steep 30 minutes. Strain and sweeten with honey. Drink at least 2 cups per day.

FENNEL

Steep 1 tsp. fennel seeds in 1 c. water, covered for a tea for asthma.

GARLIC, GLYCERIN, VINEGAR, & HONEY

For an effective cure for asthma attacks, peel 1/2 lb. garlic buds. Add equal amounts of vinegar and distilled water to cover the garlic. Use a wide-mouth jar; close it tightly, and shake well. Stand it in a cool place for four days. Shake it once or twice a day. Add 1/2 pint of glycerin. Shake the jar and let it stand another day. Strain the liquid with pressure through a sieve. Blend in 1 1/2 lbs. of honey, and place the liquid in a labeled jar. Store in a cool place. The dose is 1 tsp. with or without water every 15 minutes until the asthma spasm is controlled. Afterwards, give 1 tsp. every 2-3 hours for the rest of the day. Following the crest of the attack, give 1 tsp. three times a day.

GINGER

Ginger tea is a popular treatment for asthma. Grate 1 tsp. into boiled water.

LINSEED

A hot poultice of linseed should be applied over the front and back of the chest. This poultice may be prepared by mixing 1 cup or 16 tablespoons of the seeds with a quantity of hot water, sufficient to convert them into a moist mealy mass. This should then be applied carefully. Turpentine may also be rubbed over the chest.

MILK

Heat 1 cup of milk, add 1 tablespoon dried bee balm to the milk, and allow to steep 15 minutes. Strain and reheat. Drink several glasses a day until improvement is noticed.

CASTOR OIL & TURPENTINE

Mix together 1/2 cup of castor oil and 1/4 cup of rectified turpentine. Warm it before rubbing on the chest at bedtime. Cover with a flannel cloth to keep the area warm. Drink plenty of fluids.

ONION & OLIVE OIL

Fry onions and apply to the chest after rubbing the chest area with olive oil. Cover with a flannel cloth to keep the area warm. Place a hot water bottle over the chest area to break the congestion fast. This clears the airways and eases breathing.

ONION & HONEY

Soak thin onion slices in honey overnight. The resulting syrup is administered four times a day until an asthmatic condition improves.

POMEGRANATES

Eating pomegranates is effective against all the usual symptoms, including sore throat, cough, congestion, and fever. Available at most grocery stores.

SPINACH

50 grams of fresh leaves of spinach, and 250 ml of water should be mixed with a pinch of ammonium chloride and one teaspoonful of honey. This infusion is an effective expectorant in the treatment of bronchitis.

HIGH BLOOD PRESSURE

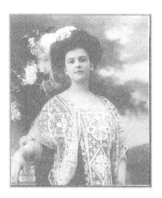

CALCIUM & POTASSIUM

Recent studies have revealed an important link between dietary calcium and potassium and hypertension. Researchers have found mat people who take potassium-rich diets have a low incidence of hypertension even if they do not control their salt intake. They have also found that people with hypertension do not seem to get much calcium in the form of dairy products. These two essential nutrients seem to help the body secrete excess sodium and are involved in important functions which control the working of the vascular system. Potassium is found in abundance in fruits and vegetables, and calcium in dairy products.

CELERY

For high blood pressure, eat celery. Celery relaxes the smooth muscle lining of blood vessels. This widens the blood vessels, and so lowers blood pressure. This should be avoided by hypertensive people who are sensitive to salt in their diets.

CELERY SEED

Celery seed may be used under the supervision of a physician as a part of a program to treat high blood pressure, congestive heart failure, or diabetes: Use 1-2 of freshly crushed seeds per cup of boiling water. Steep 10-20 minutes. Drink up to 3 c. per day.

DANDELION

Dandelion leaves are as effective as the pharmaceutical diuretics prescribed for hypertension but without the harmful side effects. Because dandelion leaves are rich in potassium, there is not the danger of creating electrolyte imbalances that can cause heart-rate disturbances. Dandelion has a bitter, but not unpleasant taste. To make a tea from dandelion, pour one cup of boiling water over two teaspoons of dried leaf, cover, and steep for 15 minutes.

GARLIC

Garlic is regarded as an effective means of lowering blood pressure. It is said to reduce spasms of the small arteries. It also slows down the pulse rate and modifies the heart rhythm, besides relieving the symptoms of dizziness, numbness, shortness of breath, and the formation of gas within the digestive tract It may be taken in the form of raw cloves or two to three capsules a day.

GOLDENSEAL

Put 1 tsp. Goldenseal in a pint of boiling water. Take a swallow of this at least six times a day. Take plenty of red clover tea, as this will purify the blood. It is good to drink this in place of water.

LEMON

Lemon is also regarded as a valuable food to control high blood pressure. It is a rich source of vitamin P which is found both in the juice and peel of the fruit this vitamin is essential for preventing capillary fragility.

LINDEN

Linden is also a mild diuretic and is excellent in combination with other herbs for treating high blood pressure. Because it helps to calm the nervous system, it is especially helpful for relieving hypertension that is related to emotional stress. Linden flower tea has a delicate, pleasant flavor. Pour one cup of boiling water over two teaspoons of dried herb, cover, and steep for 15 minutes. Strain and drink up to three cups daily.

PARSLEY

Parsley is very useful in high blood pressure. It contains elements which help maintain the blood vessels, particularly, the capillaries. It keeps the arterial system in a healthy condition. It may be taken as a beverage by simmering 20 gm of fresh parsley leaves gently in 250 ml of water for a few minutes. This may be drunk several times daily.

POTATO

Potatoes, especially in boiled form, are a valuable food for lowering blood pressure. When boiled with their skin, they absorb very little salt Thus they can form a useful addition to a salt-free diet recommended for patients with high blood pressure. Potatoes are rich in potassium but not in sodium salts. The magnesium present in the vegetable exercises beneficial effects in lowering blood pressure.

RICE

Rice has a low-fat, low-cholesterol, and low-salt content It makes a perfect diet for those hypertensive persons who have been advised salt-restricted diets. Calcium in brown rice, in particular, soothes and relaxes the nervous system and helps relieve the symptoms of high blood pressure.

VEGETABLE JUICES

Raw vegetable juices, especially carrot and spinach juices, taken separately or in combination, are also beneficial in the treatment of high blood pressure. If taken in combination, 300 ml of carrot juice and 200 ml of spinach juice should be mixed to make 500 ml or half a liter of the juice, and taken daily. If taken separately, one glass should be taken twice daily, morning and evening.

WATERMELON

Watermelon is another valuable safeguard against high blood pressure. A substance extracted from watermelon seeds is said to have a definite action in dilating the blood vessels, which results in lowering the blood pressure. The seeds, dried and roasted, should be taken in liberal quantities.

YARROW

Yarrow helps to lower blood pressure by dilating the peripheral blood vessels and also through its mild diuretic properties. It has a bitter, aromatic flavor. To make a tea, pour one cup of boiling water over two teaspoons of dried yarrow, cover, and steep for 15 minutes. Strain, and drink up to three cups a day.

THE CHRISTMAS LOCKET

Gukkie's Christian beliefs impacted me more than what I had learned in any church.

I loved her and loved the way other people loved her and decided I wanted what she had. I wasn't quite sure about how to go about getting IT yet but at age 13, I thought I would try to help someone else and see if I could discover if that was part of IT.

I became a teen counselor at a place called, "The Mansion" in San Jose, California when I was a freshman in high school. Several times a week and on weekends, I would go hang out with other teenagers, and just "be there" for anyone who needed help. I had also learned to play the guitar by this time and was writing songs.

On several occasions I played my renditions to the kids there, as well as to visiting adults. Including to, one time, the Hell's Angels. Being at the Mansion was fine except I still felt that I could be doing more on a daily basis to speed up getting IT. So, I began to keep my eyes open for anyone hurting, anywhere. Especially another kid.

I walked to and from school, and one particular day, I saw a boy walking with his head down. He was ahead of me, and I watched as he would sometimes stop, wipe his eyes, and then start walking again. This kid was considered to be the school "nerd." But, I looked at this as my big opportunity and as we walked by a park, I ran up to him.

He looked shocked that I would even talk to him. I asked him if he wanted to talk for awhile, and we wound up sitting under a tree at the park for over an hour. He told me that his parents were getting divorced, he didn't like himself and he was thinking about suicide. I must tell you, I felt more than a little over my head with his revelations. Especially the part about suicide. Scared the daylights out of me.

I told him that I would walk home with him after school every day, and we could talk more, and that I would be his friend.

It was the beginning of December and Gukkie was staying with us for the Christmas holiday season. When I got home from school one day, I rushed to her, and told her about the boy and what he had said. When I asked her what to do, she answered, "Keep your promise and talk with him every day. And pray."

I did this and two weeks later, the doorbell rang before dinner. But when I got to the door, no one was there. However when I looked down, there was a small, gift-wrapped box with my name on it. Inside I found a beautiful, gold locket in the shape of a heart. The heart had a tiny engraved cross inside and my name was engraved on the back. The accompanying note simply said, "Thank You," and was signed by the boy.

When I showed the gift to Gukkie she said, "You were doing God's work by taking time to show someone you cared, and when you do His work, the angels sing."

BURNS

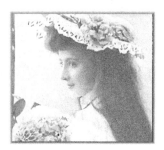

BAKING SODA & MILK

Make a pack of baking soda and milk and apply it to a sunburned face or any other area.

CUCUMBER

Cucumber juice can be rubbed into the skin to treat inflammation, burns, and sores.

GINGER

Crush fresh ginger, squeeze out the juice, and apply to the burn with a cotton ball. Stops the pain of burns instantly, reduces swelling, and helps to eliminate blistering.

LEMON & OLIVE OIL

Dip a slice of lemon in olive oil and rub it over the affected area. Helps clean the burn.

ONION

Onion juice does not necessarily relieve pain but it does act as an antiseptic.

STRAWBERRIES

To find relief from a mild sunburn, rub a cut strawberry over the face after washing to soothe the sting.

TOMATO

Cut tomato into thin slices; rub well upon hands, neck, or shoulders, and face. Let it remain for 5 minutes. Wash off with water mixed with borax (teaspoonful powdered borax to a quart of water). The application is said to bleach out sunburn and whiten the neck.

CHICKEN POX

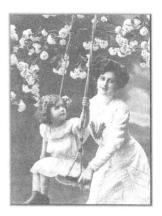

BAKING SODA

Put some baking soda in a glass of water and sponge the areas that itch. Leave the soda to dry on the skin. Controls itching.

CARROT & CORIANDER

Take a little under ½ c. of carrots and 5/8 of a c. of fresh coriander and cut into small pieces. Boil for a bit. Strain. Drink this soup once a day.

HONEY

Smear skin with honey. It is said to rid Chicken Pox within three days.

VITAMIN E OIL

Rub vitamin E oil on the skin to promote healing and prevent scarring.

CHOLESTEROL

CORIANDER SEEDS

Boil 2 Tbs. of seeds in a glass-worth of water. Cool and strain. Drink twice daily to treat high cholesterol.

LECITHIN

Take two capsules daily to treat high cholesterol.

SUNFLOWER SEEDS

Eat ½ to 1 cup daily to lower high cholesterol.

WHEAT BRAN, WHOLE CEREALS, RICE, BARLEY, RYE, LEGUMES, CARROTS, POTATOES, BEET, TURNIPS, MANGOS, GUAVAS, CABBABE, LETTUCE, CELERY & OATS

Eat often to reduce high cholesterol.

FLAVORED COLD MEDICINE

I am in a warm bedroom and the window's light sheds a soft glow on my bed and my glistening forehead. I'm 5 years old, and I have a fever...and I'm miserable. (Why is it when we're sick we feel the most alone?)

Here comes Gukkie! I can hear her voice down the hall. I'm so glad she's here! I'm so glad her plane didn't crash coming all the way from Chicago. And, I won't die.

Here she is! She's so pretty. She has a fur-thing wrapped around her neck with an animal's head that clips it together. (I wonder if the animal lived in that fur?) Oh and she smells so good. She says she doesn't wear any perfume but she must.

How can anyone smell that good just by themselves?

Oh how I love her hugs. Her cheek is so soft. And how can she be so pretty without any makeup on like Mommy wears? I don't care. I'm going to live, and that's all that matters.

Now Gukkie went to get me medicine. Oh-my-gosh, what's it going to be? What's it going to TASTE like? Uh, oh, here it comes. It's in a teaspoon, and it looks all right. Hey, it's JELLY! Is that my medicine, Gukkie? And can I have different flavors? And can I get another hug, too? Please stay with me forever.

This is one of my first vivid memories of Gukkie healing my hurts.

I remember what I felt, how she made me feel. Like Mary Poppins with a spoonful of sugar, Gukkie did more than help the medicine go down. *SHE* was the medicine.

Gukkie was intuitive and would know what was going through a sick child's mind. She knew, to a child, that the taking of medicine could be as horrible as the symptoms of the illness. To counter this, she was innovative and would think of neat and fun ways to get the "good for you stuff" to go down without a hassle. She took the time to do this.

In our age of "hurry-hurry," everyone wants a "quick fix." If you're sick, buy a bottle of stuff, take it, and hurry up and feel well enough to rush back into the fast-lane of life. Never mind that the stuff you took only lasts 3-4 hours, makes you drowsy, and only masks the symptoms. The symptoms will hide there until the real cause of the illness is treated. On top of this, no one seems to sympathize with how you feel. Because they are in too much of a hurry, too, to notice or care.

We must take the time to be nicer to ourselves and those we love. Especially in times of illness, no matter how minor that illness seems to anyone else. Any pain, as expressed by one of my father's doctors, is to be taken seriously and listened to because no one knows the depth of the pain to patient. A young child's discomfort should not be poo-pooed by adults.

It is very real to him or her. In addition, hugs go a very long way with anyone feeling crummy.

So does a Tylenol tablet smashed into jelly.

COLDS & FLU'S

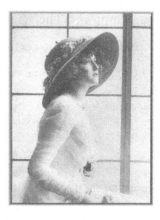

See also Bronchitis and Asthma

BASIL

Steep 5g of fresh basil in a cupful of water, then drink it to eliminate stuffiness caused by inflamed mucous membranes.

BITTER GOURD ROOT

The roots of the bitter gourd plant are used in folk medicine to cure a cold. A teaspoon of the root paste mixed with an equal quantity of honey, given once every night for a month, acts as an excellent medicine for colds.

CATNIP

Steep 1 teaspoon of catnip in 1 cup boiling water for 10 minutes. Strain and add the tea to 1 cup of cherry juice. Catnip has been used since antiquity to reduce fever by causing the patient to perspire.

CAYENNE PEPPER

A cold may generally be removed by one or two doses of the powder taken in warm water. To make a powerful liniment for sprains and congestion, gently boil 1 Tb. cayenne pepper in 1 pint of cider vinegar. Bottle the unstrained liquid while it's hot. Apply to the affected area.

CAYENNE PEPPER, SALT, & APPLE CIDER VINEGAR

For an extremely effective anti-flu remedy, grind together 2 tsp. cayenne pepper, and 1 1/2 tsp. salt to form a paste. Add 1 c. boiling water (or, better, some strong, strained chamomile tea). Steep and cool. Add 1 c. vinegar to the water. Most adults can take between a tsp. to a Tb. every half hour. If it seems too strong, dilute it. If you have a delicate digestion, take tiny doses and spread them out during the day.

CELERY & HONEY

For dizziness, mix fresh celery juice (use a food processor or blender) with honey. Celery is a strong diuretic and has a mild sedative effect.

CINNAMON

Bruise the bark and simmer in boiled water or in brandy. Take several times a day if you have been exposed to the flu.

CINNAMON, SAGE & BAY LEAVES

Said to cure a cold within 24 hours: Use a heaping teaspoon of each to a cup of boiling water; steep and drink freely.

GUKKIE'S CHICKEN SOUP FOR COLDS & SPIRITS

I t is now a well-known fact that our grandmothers knew what they were doing when they fed chicken soup to their loved ones who were under the weather. Gukkie did, and your grandmothers probably did, too.

Here is Gukkie's recipe for making her chicken soup cure-all. It is surprisingly simple to make, full of natural vitamin C and antibiotics which will help drive away the "bugs" that invade your system from time to time. This recipe also freezes and microwaves well.

Moreover, when you treat yourself to the pampering power of this soup, you will feel like you are loved. Do not ask me why this is, it just is.

INGREDIENTS

(Makes 8 servings)

1 chicken, cut up, with skin removed

3-4 medium onions, chopped

2 carrots, sliced

2 celery sticks, sliced

8 (yes, 8) cloves of garlic, minced

8 cups of water

1/2 cup brown rice (optional)

2 tablespoons minced fresh parsley

1/4 teaspoon cayenne pepper

4 teaspoons soy sauce

lemon slices (optional)

Place the chicken pieces, onions, carrots, celery, garlic and water in a large kettle.

Bring to a boil, reduce heat, and simmer.

After 50 minutes, add the rice, parsley and cayenne. Simmer an additional 30-40 minutes, until the rice is cooked. Stir in the soy sauce at the end of cooking.

To prepare for serving, allow the soup to cool slightly, and then remove the bones from the chicken, returning the chicken meat to the stock. Reheat before serving. Place a lemon slice on top of each bowlful of soup, if desired. Makes about 10 cups.

COMFREY

Chop several leaves of comfrey and add 1/2 cup of elderberries. Add 1 cup of honey and 1 cup of water. Simmer for 30 minutes. Strain and take as needed to produce perspiration and reduce fever. The comfrey leaves produce an aspirin-like substance and help to ease the discomforts of a cold, as well as soothe inflamed mucous membranes of the throat. Comfrey is considered a demulcent and an expectorant. The elderberries serve as a diuretic to flush the system.

COMFREY #2

If congestion is present, try this comfrey recipe. Add 2 tablespoons of comfrey root (cut up fine) to 1 pint of water. Bring to a boil and then simmer for 30 minutes. Strain and sweeten. Take this 3-4 times daily by the cup. Comfrey reduces the inflammation in the bronchial and alimentary system. It acts as an emollient, demulcent, and expectorant. Not bad, for one simple herb. It also has pain-relieving properties, so you are more comfortable while fighting a cold.

CORN HUSKS

Boil 8 corn husks in 4 cups of water for about 30 minutes. Strain and drink. Said to relieve headaches and stuffiness of the nose during a cold.

GARLIC

Chew 3 raw cloves to ward off a cold or flu, or will lessen the symptoms if in progress. Odor-free garlic tablets work almost as well.

GARLIC SOUP: GARLIC, CHICKEN SOUP OR BOUILLON, & EGGS

A delicious recipe for a cold or flu! Cut up half-a-dozen cloves of garlic and saute' in oil, being careful not to let them burn. Add a quart of stock (such as beef), and let it come to a boil for just a few moments. Then lower the heat. Separate two eggs and add the whites to the hot liquid, stirring rapidly. Mix the yolks with two Tbs. of vinegar and then pour them in. Add salt and pepper if you want and some croutons, if handy. It works and it's delicious.

GARLIC SOUP #2

Garlic soup is an old remedy to reduce the severity of a cold, and should be taken once daily. The soup can be prepared by boiling three or four cloves of chopped garlic in a cup of water. Garlic contains antiseptic and antispasmodic properties, besides several other medicinal virtues. The oil contained in this vegetable helps to open up the respiratory passages. In soup form, it flushes out all toxins from the system and thus helps bring down fever. Five drops of garlic oil combined with a teaspoon of onion juice, and diluted in a cup of water, should be drunk two to three times a day. This has also been found to be very effective in the treatment of common cold.

GINGER & HONEY

Use ginger tea sweetened with honey to break up a cold; grate 1 tsp. ginger root in boiling water. Take it of the heat, cover, and steep for 10-15 minutes. Add honey to taste.

GINGER ROOT & MILK

Boil fresh ginger root in milk and inhale the vapors. To prevent future colds, chew a small piece of ginger root before meals.

GINGER TEA

Ginger is another excellent remedy for colds and coughs. About 10 grams of ginger should be cut into small pieces and boiled in a cup of water. It should then be strained and half a teaspoon of sugar added to it. This decoction should be drunk while hot. Ginger tea, prepared by adding a few pieces of ginger into boiled water before adding tea leaves, is also an effective remedy for colds and for fevers resulting from cold. It may be taken twice daily.

LEMON

Before bedtime, sip one or more glasses of hot water with lemon juice. This has vitamin C to fight the cold, and the juice helps to ease sore throat pain. Lemon is the most important among the many home remedies for common cold. It is beneficial in all types of cold with fever. Vitamin C-rich lemon juice increases body resistance, decreases toxicity and reduces the duration of the illness. One lemon should be diluted in a glass of warm water, and a teaspoon of honey should be added to it This should be taken once or twice daily.

LEMONADE

Heat a glass of lemonade and add honey to sweeten. This is a good recipe if you have a cold with a fever. It relaxes you and is helpful in relieving discomfort.

MILK

At the onset of a cold, add 1/2 teaspoon each of cinnamon and ginger to 1 cup of scalded milk. Add 1 tablespoon of honey and drink while hot. Very soothing and stimulating.

MULLEIN FLOWER TEA

Mullein flower tea has a pleasant taste and is good to soothe inflamed conditions of the mucous membrane lining the throat. Additionally, Mullein flower tea relieves coughing. Put a small handful of the mullein flowers in 1 pint of boiling water. Allow to steep 15 minutes. Strain and sweeten with honey.

MUSTARD POWDER

Make into a paste with flour and warm water and apply in a cloth to aid congestion. The powder may also be added to foot baths to help decongest the nasal passages.

ONION

George Washington's favorite cold remedy was to eat a hot roasted onion just before going to bed.

SPECIAL COLD REMEDY

Pour 1 gallon of water in a large pan, adding 1/3 cup softened ginger root, 3 cups of honey, and 1 cup seedless raisins. Bring to a boil and simmer for about an hour. The top will have to be skimmed every once in a while. Cool, strain, and place in a tightly closed container overnight in the refrigerator. The next day, squeeze 6 lemons and 4 oranges and add the juice to the mixture. Mix well and drink 2-3 glasses per day. This will get rid of symptoms pretty fast and clean the system.

TERRIFIC TONIC

This was the best place I could find to put this wonderful, cure-all tonic. This tonic relieves the symptoms of colds, flu's, hangovers, nausea and stomachache. It takes many ingredients, most found easily at a health food store or herb shop and well-worth the effort to make:

2 pints Madeira wine

1 sprig wormwood

1 sprig rosemary

1 small bruised nutmeg

1 inch bruised gingerroot

1 inch bruised cinnamon bark

12 large organic raisins

Pour off about an ounce of the wine. Place herbs in the wine. Cork the bottle tightly. Place the bottle in a cool, dark place for a week or two. Strain off the herbs. Combine this medicated wine with a fresh bottle of Madeira. Mix thoroughly. Sip a small amount at a time whenever needed. You may also use the medicated wine alone, undiluted with the un-medicated wine to help settle the stomach, get energy, and well, make you feel much better. CAUTION: too much of this can make you feel so much better you could be seeing cross-eyed.

Foot Baths for Colds

Put 1 1/4 cup of dried mustard in 8 cups of boiling water and boil for 10 minutes. Add this liquid to a foot bath to treat colds and respiratory problems.

Royal Mix for Severe Colds

Mix 1 cup each of dried white yarrow, spearmint, sage, catnip, horehound, verbena, and pennyroyal. Pour 2 cups of boiling water over 2 1/2 tablespoons of the herb mix. Cover and let stand 10 minutes. Strain and sweeten. Reheat and drink 1 cup every couple of hours. Use more often if sweating is desired.

Sweeten Breath during Colds

Chew fresh parsley during a cold. This not only freshens the breath during a cold, but rids the mouth of any bad odors anytime. Parsley also gives you the extra vitamins you need while suffering through a cold.

COLITIS

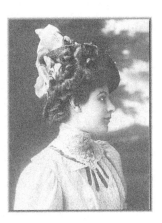

APPLES

Steamed apples promote the healing of ulcerative lesions.

APPLE CIDER VINEGAR

Dip a flannel cloth in apple cider vinegar and place on abdomen. Cover with plastic wrap and leave on at least 4 hours.

BANANA

Eat one or two ripe bananas every day to promote the healing process. Bananas are also a slight laxative.

BUTTERMILK

Drink one glass of buttermilk per day as an effective treatment for colitis.

EPSOM SALTS

Mix 2 c. of Epsom salts in 2 c. of water. Saturate a flannel cloth in the solution and place over the abdomen. Put a heating pad or hot water bottle on top to keep warm for 3-4 hours.

RICE

Mix rice with a glass of buttermilk and ripe banana to make a thick cereal. Eat twice a day.

CONSTIPATION

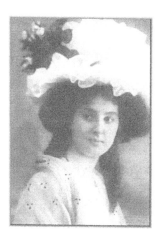

BASIL & OLIVE OIL

Find a clear-glass container that has a tightly-fitting screw top. Fill the container with roughly chopped basil leaves. Cover with olive oil, and let the jar stand in bright sunlight for 3 weeks. After 3 weeks, strain the oil into another jar full of chopped basil. After 6 weeks, the oils is ready to be used. Take 1 tsp. to calm stomach cramps after a meal or to ease constipation.

BANANA OR DRY FIGS

Eat a very ripe banana or some dried figs first thing in the morning on an empty stomach.

COFFEE

Drink a strong cup of caffeinated or decaffeinated coffee first thing in the morning on an empty stomach as a quick treatment for occasional constipation.

GRAPEFRUIT JUICE OR MILK

Make it a habit to drink grapefruit juice or milk daily to avoid constipation.

HONEY

Take by the teaspoon as needed.

LEMON JUICE

Mix 1 teaspoon each of lemon juice and olive oil. Take on a daily basis.

MUSTARD SEEDS

Eat whole mustard seeds to treat indigestion and nausea. The seeds are also an effective laxative.

ORANGE

Orange is also beneficial in the treatment of constipation. Taking one or two oranges at bedtime and again on rising in the morning is an excellent way of stimulating the bowels. The general stimulating influence of orange juice excites peristaltic activity and helps prevent the accumulation of food residue in the colon.

PAPAYA AND FIGS

Other fruits specific for constipation are papaya and figs. Half a medium-sized papaya should be eaten at breakfast to act as a laxative. Both fresh and dry figs have a laxative effect Four or five dry figs should be soaked overnight in a little water and eaten in the morning.

PEAR

Pears are beneficial in die treatment of constipation. Patients suffering from chronic constipation should adopt an exclusive diet of this fruit or its juice for a few days, but in ordinary cases, a medium-sized pear taken after dinner or with breakfast will have the desired effect.

PRUNES

Self-explanatory. (Now they're put out with neat flavors like "orange zest and cinnamon," etc.)

SPINACH

Among the vegetables, spinach has been considered to be the most vital food for the entire digestive tract from tune immemorial. Raw spinach contains the finest organic material for the cleansing, reconstruction, and regeneration of the intestinal tract. Raw spinach juice—100 ml, mixed with an equal quantity of water and taken twice dairy, will cure the most aggravated cases of constipation within a few days.

SUNFLOWER SEEDS & HONEY

Take 30g shelled sunflower seeds, crush them, add 1 c. boiling water, and stir in some honey. Drink this combination in the morning and evening. Also chew 90g of walnuts.

COUGHS

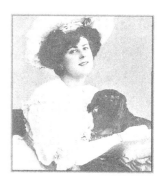

ALMONDS

Almonds are useful for dry coughs. 7 almonds should be soaked in water overnight and the brown skin removed. They should then be ground well to form a fine paste. A quantity of 20 grams each of butter and sugar should be added to the paste. This paste should be taken in the morning and evening.

ANISEED COUGH TEA

Aniseed is another effective remedy for a hard dry cough with difficult expectoration. It breaks up the mucus. A tea is made from this spice and taken regularly.

CHERRY COUGH SYRUP

Place 2 cups of cherries in a pan and add just enough water to cover. Add several lemon slices and 2 cups of honey. Simmer the mixture until cherries are soft. Remove from heat. Remove the lemon slices and the cherry pits from the mixture. Refrigerate and take several tablespoons as needed for coughing.

FIGS

Boil 6 figs in milk for 10 minutes. Take a cupful several times a day.

GARLIC COUGH SYRUP

Remedy for bronchial complaints ranging from bronchitis to asthma. Slice 2 ½ cups of fresh garlic into 4 c. of water. Bruise 2 Tbs. each of caraway and fennel seeds. Add to garlic water. Boil this mixture until garlic is soft. Let stand 12-14 hours in a very tightly closed container. Measure the mixture at the end of 14 hours and add an equal amount of cider vinegar. Bring again to a boil, adding enough sugar to make a syrup. Take 1 tsp. as needed for cough.

GARLIC & BRANDY

Make a garlic tincture by placing three to four peeled buds in brandy. Steep this in a dark closet for 14 days. Use several drops at a time, several times a day for coughs or asthma. Garlic is an exceptional cleanser for the body and has antimicrobial action similar to other antibiotics.

GARLIC, FENNEL, CARAWAY, VINEGAR, & SUGAR

Considered by many herbalists to be a sovereign remedy for bronchial complaints ranging from asthma to bronchitis is Garlic Syrup: Slice 1 lb. fresh garlic bulbs and boil them until soft in 1 quart of water, adding 1/2 oz. each of bruised fennel and caraway seed. Let this stand for 12 hours in a closely covered container before straining. Add to the resultant liquor an equal quantity of vinegar, bringing it back to the boil, and add enough sugar to make it into the consistency of a syrup. One spoonful of syrup may be taken each morning and whenever necessary.

GARLIC POWDER & SUGAR

Mix 2 tsp. of garlic powder with some sugar and eat.

GRAPE JUICE

Grapes are one of the most effective home remedies for the treatment of coughs. Grapes tone up the lungs and act as an expectorant, relieving a simple cold and cough in a couple of days. A cup of grape juice mixed with a teaspoon of honey provides relief.

HORSERADISH

Scrape some fresh root into a clean bowl. Cover the grated root with sugar and turn frequently for a day until there is a layer of syrup at the bottom of the bowl. Drain the syrup off into a clean bottle. Take 3 times a day, 1 Tb. at a time.

MULLEIN AND MALLOW FLOWERS

Mix 1/4 cup each of mullein and mallow flowers. (Either the mullein leaves or flowers can be used.) Add 1 tablespoon of herb mixture to 1 cup of boiling water. Strain and add several cloves and 1 teaspoon of lemon juice. Sweeten with honey. Loosens chest congestion and promotes discharge of mucus (expectorant).

MUSTARD POWDER

Make mustard powder into a thick paste. Heat and spread on a cloth, and apply to the chest. Decreases congestion in the chest area.

ONION

The use of raw onion is valuable in a cough. The onion should be chopped fine and the juice extracted from it. One teaspoon of the onion juice should be mixed with one teaspoon of honey and kept for four or five hours. It makes an excellent cough syrup. Take twice daily to help remove phlegm. Additionally, a medium-sized onion can be crushed and the juice of one lemon added to it; add one cup of boiling water poured over it. A teaspoon of honey can be added for taste. Take 2-3 times per day.

OREGANO

For coughs and to treat a cold, use 1-2 tsp. dried herb per cup of boiling water. Steep 10 minutes. Drink up to 3 cups a day. Will loosen phlegm and make it easier to cough up.

PARSLEY COUGH TEA

This is good to use for a persistent, stubborn cough. Pour 2 ½ cups of boiling water over 2 Tbs. of dried agrimony flowers or leaves, and 1 Tbs. dried parsley. Cover and steep until cool. Strain. Use as a gargle to soothe sore throats. To stop persistent coughs, take 2-3 Tbs. morning and evening.

RAISINS

A sauce prepared from raisins is also useful for coughs. The sauce is prepared by grinding 100 gm of raisins with water. About 100 gm of sugar should be mixed with it and the mixture heated. When the mixture acquires a sauce-like consistency, it needs to be preserved. Take 20 grams at bedtime daily.

RED CABBAGE & HONEY

Liquefy a red cabbage in the blender. The juice is strained and weighed, and half its weight in honey is added. The mixture is simmered over a low heat until syrupy. Take several doses of 2 tsp. each in quick succession.

RED ONION, SALT, & BUTTER

Make an onion broth: Cut up a large red onion and add a pint of cold water, a pinch of salt, and a pat of butter, and simmer until onion is soft. Place the broth in a bowl, and eat it as hot as possible. This also helps to induce perspiration (to lower a fever), releases toxins, and relieves chest congestion.

THYME COUGH SYRUP

Pour 2 cups boiling water over 2 tablespoons of dried thyme. Cool to room temperature. Strain and add 1 cup of honey. Shake to mix well. Keep refrigerated. Take 1 tablespoon several times a day for sore throats, colds and coughing.

TURMERIC

The root of the turmeric plant is useful in a dry cough. The root should be roasted and powdered. This powder should be taken in three gram doses twice daily, in the morning and evening.

TURNIPS

Boil good turnips in water and having expressed the juice, mix with it as much finely powdered sugar candy (table sugar) as will bring it into a kind of syrup, of which let the patient swallow a little as slowly as he can from time to time.

CUTS & SCRAPES

BAY LEAVES

For first aid, apply some freshly crushed leaves to minor cuts and scrapes.

CARROT

Boil carrots, mash them, and apply them to sores to extract pus and heal the area. Carrots are a very strong antiseptic.

CAYENNE PEPPER

A tiny bit of cayenne pepper can stop bleeding from a cut.

GARLIC

Raw cloves of garlic are placed at the edges of a wound to promote healing. Garlic is an antiseptic, along with being a natural and effective antibiotic.

DIABETES

BITTER GOURD

Take the juice of four or five Bitter Gourd every morning on an empty stomach. The seeds can also be added to food in powdered form. Said to be proven to be beneficial in controlling diabetes.

FENUGREEK

Take 25-50 gm daily. Found to be effective in the treatment of diabetes.

STRAWBERRY LEAVES

Place 4-5 fresh leaves in 1 c. of boiling water. Steep 15 minutes. Strain and drink.

VEGETABLES

Eat plenty of cucumber, onion, string beans, and garlic to treat diabetes.

RAGGEDY ANN & PINK ELEPHANTS

When I was about two or three years old, I had a pink elephant. It was stuffed (I loved the trunk), and had the most enchanting "carpet" on its back. This elephant was reminiscent of "Arabian Nights" as this covering was adorned with sequins, beads, small mirrors, and pearls of all colors.

But most of all, it had been made by Gukkie.

I had that elephant until I was 16 and then I think it got lost in a move.

Other relatives in our family possess Gukkie's adorable re-creations of Raggedy Ann and Andy. I would give my right arm to have one of those sets since I've missed my "ele-ele." Sound crazy? It isn't when you stop to consider who's BEHIND these creations.

I think that part of the reason we, even as adults, grow so attached to "things" is because these things provide a connection to those we love. And, Gukkie was a pro at keeping her connections to those she cared about locked in solid. She never had to say anything to remind us of this.

If Gukkie wasn't concocting some remedial brew for an illness, she was creating another sort of treatment for the healing of the heart; a doll or stuffed animal. And, she certainly left her mark by doing this. You see she knew that long after the illness was gone, she had made sure that she left a reminder of her caring for you. The doll or animal stayed at your side to remind you of someone's thoughtful, tender loving care.

There are many different kinds of remedies for various conditions, illnesses, and ailments. The treatments that seem to work the best and have long-lasting benefits are made with love. That sounds so corny, but there isn't any other way to put it.

The lesson from Gukkie is: leave your mark. Never be ashamed to show where you've been in this life. Good or bad, it's all for the purpose of growth as a SPIRIT.

Be an on-going presence in this world through the lives of others long after you're gone.

To this day, I'm sure that Gukkie continues to make the angels sing.

Gukkie took roads that others wished to follow.

Lucky for the many who had known her, Gukkie thought enough about us to leave her footprints behind. But then she would say that those footprints were never hers alone.

DIARRHEA

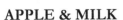

ALLSPICE

Put a pinch of allspice in 1 cup of warm water. Add honey and drink after every bowel movement.

APPLE

Peel, core, and puree an apple in the blender. Grate if you do not have a blender. Give 1 apple every 2 hours while withholding all other food during treatment.

APPLE & MILK

Simmer 1 pared apple in 1 cup of milk until very soft. Put apple and milk mixture in the blender and blend until smooth. Drink 1/2 cup after every bowel movement until relief is obtained.

BUTTERMILK

Buttermilk is one of the most effective home remedies in the treatment of diarrhea. Buttermilk is the residual milk left after the fat has been removed from curd by churning. It helps overcome harmful intestinal flora. The acid in the buttermilk also fights germs and bacteria. Buttermilk may be taken with a pinch of salt three or four times a day for controlling diarrhea.

CARROTS

Cooked carrots are an especially effective remedy for infant diarrhea.

CARROT SOUP

Carrot soup is another effective home remedy for diarrhea. It supplies water to combat dehydration; replenishes sodium, potassium, phosphorus, calcium, sulphur, and magnesium; supplies pectin; and coats the intestine to allay inflammation. It also checks the growth of harmful intestinal bacteria and prevents vomiting. Half a kilogram of carrots may be cooked in 150 ml of water until they become soft. The pulp should be strained and enough boiled water added to it to make a liter. Three-quarters of a tablespoon of salt may be added. This soup should be given in small amounts to the patient every half an hour.

CEREALS, BANANAS, TAPIOCA, & POTATOES

Here we go again, with the potato business. Maybe Gukkie gave them to my mom and aunt on a regular basis for a reason. Use any of these items to help cure diarrhea.

FENUGREEK

Fenugreek leaves are useful in diarrhea. One teaspoon of seeds which have been boiled and fried in butter should be taken with a cup of buttermilk twice daily. They are valuable in allaying biliousness. The seeds are also beneficial in the treatment of this disease.

GARLIC & BROWN SUGAR

Peel and crush 2 cloves of garlic, add 2 tsp. of brown sugar, then pour in about ½ c. of boiling water. Drink 2-3 times daily.

GINGER

In case of diarrhea caused by indigestion, dry or fresh ginger is very useful A piece of dry ginger should be powdered along with a crystal of rock salt, and quarter of a teaspoon of this powder should be taken with small piece of jaggery. It will bring quick relief as ginger, being carminative, aids digestion by stimulating the gastrointestinal tract.

MINT

Mint juice is also beneficial in the treatment of diarrhea. One teaspoon of fresh mint juice, mixed with a teaspoon each of lime juice and honey, can be given thrice daily with excellent results in the treatment of this disease.

NUTMEG

Heat 1 cup of milk. Add 1 teaspoon of nutmeg. Stir well and drink warm. Do this every hour until relief is obtained. Honey may be added if desired.

POMEGRANATE

The pomegranate has proved beneficial in the treatment of diarrhea on account of its astringent properties. If the patient develops weakness due to profuse and continuous purging, he should repeatedly be given about 50 ml of pomegranate juice to drink. This will control the diarrhea.

RICE

Cooked rice is useful in controlling irritable diarrhea.

SWEET POTATOES

Eat boiled sweet potatoes seasoned with salt and pepper before bedtime to cure chronic diarrhea.

TOMATO

A glass of fresh tomato juice, mixed with a pinch of salt and pepper, taken in the morning, also proves beneficial.

TURMERIC

Turmeric has proved to be another valuable home remedy for diarrhea. It is a very useful intestinal antiseptic. It is also a gastric stimulant and tonic. One teaspoon of fresh turmeric rhizome juice or one teaspoon of dry rhizome powder may be taken in one cup of buttermilk or plain water.

EARACHES

CARAWAY, BREAD, & BRANDY

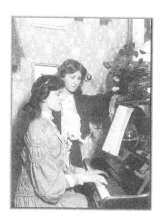

Heat an unsliced bread loaf in the oven. Throw away the crust and pound together the soft bread and a handful of bruised caraway seeds. Add some hot brandy and apply the paste as a hot poultice to the ear or any other inflammation.

CHAMOMILE

Steep 1-2 tsp. flowers in boiling water for 10-15 minutes. Strain out the water, and apply the hot flowers in a cloth for alleviation of the earache.

GARLIC

Place a peeled clove of garlic in the ear(s): The clove is held in place with a piece of cotton. Do not leave in for long periods of time; alternate ears so irritations don't occur. In fact, a better alternative is to place slivers of garlic in gauze, then place in the ear(s).

GARLIC OIL

Crush a few cloves of garlic into some olive oil and let it sit for a few days at room temperature. Stain this mixture and refrigerate. Warm it to room temperature before use. Place a few drops of the oil in the ear canal, then plug loosely with sterile cotton or gauze. Do not use this remedy if there is any ear discharge or any indication that the eardrum is perforated.

ONION

Roast an onion and after it cools, wrap it in a piece of cloth and place over the ear. Continue procedure until the pain stops.

VICS VAPORUB

Menthol.

This particular stuff has been a favorite of "folk medicine practitioners" for many years in treating colds, asthma, and other breathing problems.

Do you remember the gooey stuff being smeared all over your chest, smudged under your nose, and glopped into any other orifice deemed worthy of its benefits? Did you get the hot-wash-cloth-on-the-chest-over-the-goo routine?

When it came to colds, Gukkie was the first to produce Vics, Eucalyptus, hot small towel, humidifier if handy, and of course, a hot potato smothered in butter. And---her chicken soup.

Now, I'm not endorsing any particular "mentholated" product, and Gukkie wouldn't either. The idea is to open your breathing cavities and cleanse them of the yucky gooey stuff, so that you can breathe.

Personally, I'm in love with Eucalyptus oil. Even allergies respond to its "opening of the breathing passages" abilities. You can even breathe the stuff right from the bottle, and you're "open." Gukkie was also fond of burning pine candles, and I've learned to burn ANY candle with some Eucalyptus oil dropped on it.

1 tablespoon of Eucalyptus oil can also be put into the water of a humidifier. 3 cups of pine needles in 2 cups of water can be boiled down to 1 cup of liquid and added to the water. Any of it can be added to your bath water or smeared on your person. And then WRAP UP! I can still hear Gukkie's words echo that to this day when I have a cold or flu. That and to keep socks on my feet at all times.

And, "air out the house" by keeping a couple of windows open or even cracked even if it's storming outside. BUT keep the sick person away from a direct draft from any such opening.

And give a lot of hugs to the ailing patient. Gukkie did.

Remember, hugs contain more healing powers than any herb or drug.

ECZEMA

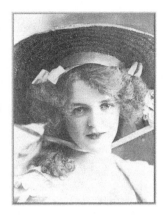

CANTALOUPE (MUSK MELON)

Eat three melon-balls' worth for three days. After that add one ball to the number daily until it is enough to satisfy hunger. Eat for 40 days.

LEMON JUICE

Apply lemon juice to the area and allow drying before bed. Leave on overnight. Helps to heal the skin and acts as an antiseptic if the area is inflamed.

MANGO

Simmer the pulp and skin of a mango in 1 c. of water. Strain and apply liberally as a lotion to the affected areas several times daily.

POTATO

Grate a raw potato and apply as a poultice to relieve the itching instantly.

EYE PROBLEMS

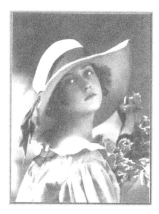

ALMONDS

Grind several kernels finely with a touch of pepper in half a cup of water sweetened with 1 tsp. of sugar. Helps the eyes regain their vigor after drinking.

CARROT

Eating several raw carrots or drinking carrot juice is beneficial treating cataracts.

CORIANDER

Boil a handful of dried coriander in 1 c. of water. Cool. Use as an eyewash to relieve the burning and itching of red eye (Conjunctivitis). Do not use if you have asthma or chronic bronchitis.

GARLIC

Eat 2-3 raw cloves should be slowly chewed daily to clean the crystalline lens of the eye and help relieve cataracts.

HONEY (unprocessed)

Put a few drops in the eye to treat cataracts.

HONEY AND APPLE CIDER VINEGAR

Mix 2 tsp. each of honey and apple cider vinegar in a glass of water. Drink with every meal to retard cataract growth as well as to prevent cataracts.

CUCUMBER

Pink eyes, sunburn, and eyestrain may all be relieved by the application of cooling and refreshing cucumber slices to the closed eyes.

HONEY

Dissolve honey in warm water and drip into irritated eyes. Then soak a linen compress in the solution and hold it over each eye for 10 or 15 minutes.

HYDROMEL: HONEY & WATER

For Hydromel, an eye lotion, simmer a cup of water and a tsp. of honey for 5 minutes. Dip a cloth in the liquid and apply to the <u>closed</u> eye.

POTATO

(Is there no end to the potato thing? Guess we should always have a few of them around.) Make a poultice out of scraped raw potatoes and apply to closed eyes to soothe them. Warmed, this poultice helps to cure a sty.

STALE BREAD

Take a slice of stale bread, cut as thin as possible, toast both sides well, but do not burn it. When cold, soak it in cold water, then put it between a piece of old linen and apply to irritated eyes, changing when it gets warm.

TEA BAGS

Apply cooled tea bags to itching, reddened eyes to provide almost instant relief. For a sty, place tea bags on the eyelid while still warm.

TOMATOES

Eat 1 or 2 tomatoes first thing in the morning on an empty stomach to relieve bloodshot eyes.

FATIGUE

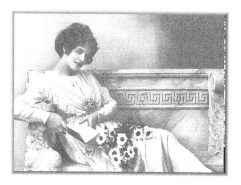

B VITAMINS

The patient should also take natural vitamins and mineral supplements as an effective assurance against nutritional deficiencies as such deficiencies cause fatigue. Lack of pantothenic acid, a B vitamin, in particular, leads to extreme fatigue as deficiency of this vitamin is associated with exhaustion of the adrenal glands. A daily dosage of 30 mg of pantothenic acid or vitamin B5 is recommended. However, the entire B complex group should be taken, with the recommended quantity of pantothenic acid, so as to avoid imbalance of some of the other B vitamins. In fact the entire B complex group protects nerves and increases energy by J helping to nourish and regulate glands. Foods rich in vitamin B are brewer's yeast, wheat germ, rice polishing, and liver.

CEREAL SEEDS

The patient suffering from fatigue should eat nutritious foods which supply energy to the body. Cereal seeds in their natural state relieve fatigue and provide energy. These 1 cereal seeds are corn seeds, wheat seeds, rye seeds, maize seeds, barley seeds, and oat seeds. They must be freshly milled. In uncooked cereals we have a perfect food for perfect health which contains the essential vitamins and energy creators. In addition to cereal seeds, fresh raw nuts should be taken directly.

DATES

Dates are an effective home remedy for fatigue and those suffering from tiredness should consume them regularly. Five to seven dates should be soaked overnight in half a cup of water and crushed in the morning in the same water after removing the seeds. This water with the essence of the dates should be taken at least twice a week.

GINSENG

Ginseng (panax ginseng and Panax quinquefolium) is said to replace lost chi, or life energy, and numerous research studies support its reputation as a restorative tonic. Ginseng helps the body adapt more easily to physical and emotional stressors by strengthening the function of the adrenal glands. Ginseng can sometimes cause overstimulation, with symptoms such as headaches or irritability. If this occurs, cut back on the amount you are taking and use American ginseng (panax quinquefolium) because it is less stimulating than the Chinese variety.

Ginseng is best used cyclically to prevent the problem of over stimulation-take it for two weeks, and then take a two-week break before resuming the dosage. For best results, buy an extract standardized for ginsenosides, which are considered to be the active compounds. Ginseng supplements vary widely in concentration-follow the manufacturer's instructions and decrease the dosage if necessary.

GRAPEFRUIT

Grapefruit has been found valuable in allaying fatigue. Taking a glass of grapefruit and lemon juice in equal parts is an excellent way of dispelling fatigue and general tiredness after a day's work.

HO SHOU WU

Ho shou wu (Polygonum multiflorum) also called fo-ti, is a Chinese herb that is similar to ginseng in its effects, but milder. It is considered to be a beneficial tonic for the reproductive organs, liver, and kidneys, all which are critical for energy and vitality. Ho shou wu is also a tonic for the thyroid gland which helps to regulate metabolism and energy. Because ho shou wu is not an immediate energizer, you need to take it over a long period (usually at least a couple of months) to feel the effects. Take one-half teaspoon of liquid extract two to three times daily in a small amount of warm water.

MINERALS

Minerals are also important. Potassium is essential for protection against fatigue. Green leafy vegetables, oranges, potatoes and lentils are rich in this mineral. Calcium is essential for relaxation and is beneficial in cases of insomnia and tension, both of which can lead to fatigue. Milk and milk products, green vegetables, sesame seeds, almonds, oats, and walnuts ate rich sources of calcium. Sodium and zinc are also beneficial in the treatment of fatigue. Foods such as celery, cucumber, lettuce, and apples are good sources of sodium; while legumes, whole grain products and pumpkin seeds contain ample quantities of zinc.

SIBERIAN GINSENG

Siberian Gingseng (Eleutherococcus senticosus), although not a true ginseng, has very similar properties and is a whole-body tonic that helps to restore healthy adrenal functioning. It significantly increases energy for both physical and mental tasks and bolsters resistance to stress. Taking Siberian ginseng regularly helps to increase both physical and psychological well-being. Take 250 milligrams two times a day of an extract standardized for eleutherosides, which are considered to be the active ingredient. For best results, take Siberian ginseng in cycles of two months, followed by a two-week break before resuming the dosage.

FEVER

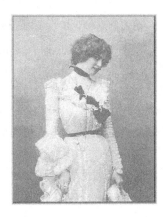

APPLES

Steep apple peelings for a few minutes in boiling water and add lemon, orange juice, peppermint, or other flavor as desired. Peelings may be used fresh or dried in the oven for future use.

APRICOT

A cup of fresh juice of apricots mixed with one teaspoon of glucose or honey is a very cooling drink during fevers. It quenches the thirst and eliminates the waste products from the body. It tones up the eyes, stomach, liver, heart, and nerves by supplying vitamins and minerals.

BAKING SODA

Fever patients can be made cool and comfortable by frequent spongings with soda water.

CAYENNE PEPPER

Add a pinch or more of the pepper to any herbal drink.

FENUGREEK

A tea made from fenugreek seeds is equal in value to quinine in reducing fevers. This tea should be taken twice daily. It is particularly valuable as a cleansing and soothing 4 Fenugreek seeds, when moistened with water, become slightly mucilaginous, and hence, the tea made from diem has the power to dissolve a sticky substance like mucus.

GRAPEFRUIT

The juice of grapefruit is a valuable diet in all fevers. It quenches thirst and removes the burning sensation produced by the fever. Half a glass of grapefruit juice should be taken with an equal quantity of water.

GRAPES

Grapes and greatly diluted grape juice are very restorative, and act on the kidneys to increase the flow of urine. This is useful in reducing fever.

HOLY BASIL

The leaves of holy basil are one of the most effective of several home remedies in the treatment of common fever. A decoction made of about 12 grams of these leaves, boiled in half a liter of water, should be administered twice daily with half a cup of milk, one teaspoon of sugar and a quarter teaspoon of powdered cardamom. This will bring down the temperature.

LEMON

Take a fresh, unpeeled, washed lemon, cut it into thin slices. Add 3 cups of water and simmer the slices in a non-aluminum pot. Reduce the juice to 1 cup. Stain and drink to cool down the body and fever.

ORANGE

Orange is an excellent food in all types of fever when the digestive power of the body is seriously hampered. The patient suffers from blood poisoning called toxemia, and the lack of saliva results in the coating of his tongue, often destroying his thirst for water as well as his desire for food. The agreeable flavor of orange juice helps greatly in overcoming these drawbacks. Orange juice is the ideal liquid food in fevers. It provides energy, increases urinary output, and promotes body resistance against infections.

RAISINS

The use of an extract from raisins is beneficial in the treatment of common fever. This extract is prepared by soaking 25 raisins in half a cup of water and then crushing them in the same water. They are then strained and the skin is discarded. The raisin water thus prepared becomes a tonic. Half a teaspoon of lime juice, added to the extract will enhance its taste and usefulness. It will act as a medicine in fevers, and should be taken twice daily.

RICE

Cook rice with a lot of water and drink the strained water. This is a nutritious drink for feverish conditions or for an inflammation of the lungs or bowels.

SAFFRON

A tea made from saffron is another effective home remedy for fever. This tea is prepared by putting half a teaspoon of saffron in 30 ml of boiling water. The patient should be given a teaspoon of this tea every hour until the temperature returns to normal.

HOT POTATOES & GOODIE PLATTERS

I call them "goodie platters." My mom and aunt call them "plates."

Whatever you want to call them, Gukkie started it.

My mom and my aunt have told me delightful stories about coming home from school in Denver where they grew up. It would be snowing and icy cold, and Gukkie never failed to have a hot potato waiting for them in the oven. Later in the evening, before bed, they would ask Gukkie for a "plate." This plate was never quite the same but it always contained a scrumptious assortment of odds and ends that Gukkie would dig out of the cupboard and refrigerator.

Gukkie lived with my mom and my aunt for most of their years growing up. This was due to the fact that my grandmother (their mother), was extremely ill with tuberculosis and was in a hospital for the treatment of T.B. Gukkie, knowing these girls needed every extra help in their own lives, literally moved into the situation to be there for them and their father, her son-in-law.

Gukkie not only tended to the house and the meals, but enriched the lives of the little girls who needed a mother's love. She didn't stop with doing only what was needed or required by the family, but invented small, yet meaningful, ways to make life more interesting and fun. And surprises were at the top of her list to accomplish this.

A "plate" could contain quartered apples and oranges, a handful of potato chips, celery and peanut butter, and cookies one night. There could be a couple of scoops of Jell-O, crackers with spread, and popcorn another. You just never knew. It was such a simple, yet thoughtful gesture that, to this day, my mom and aunt recall those "plates" with very fond memories.

In this case, we're dealing with time as the most critical factor. The time it took Gukkie to make the lives of those around her more fulfilled, she initiated the use of these "plates." It took her time to dream them up and make them.

Nevertheless, they are so remembered.

Today, I make "goodie platters" for my own family and every time I do, I think of the woman who started it all…just as I recall many of her loving-kindness and gestures for me and others generations later.

GALL BLADDER

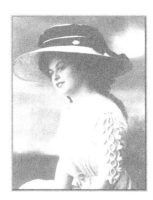

BEETS

Combine equal parts of beet, carrot, and cucumber juice and drink a glass twice a day. Said to be one of the best cleansers of the gall bladder.

LEMON JUICE

Take 4 Tbs. every morning on an empty stomach. Continue for at least 1 week to get results.

PEAR

Drink or eat pear daily for an excellent remedy for gall bladder problems.

SUNFLOWER OR OLIVE OIL

Take 2 Tbs. first thing in the morning followed by ½ c. of grapefruit or lemon juice. Continue for several days or weeks as needed.

HANGOVERS

SPINACH

Simmer large quantities of spinach (including roots and heads) over low heat for 2-3 hours. Drink warm or cool.

STRAWBERRIES

Eat 8-10 fresh strawberries. (I know this works but who is going to DRIVE to get them?)

SUGAR CUBE, CLOVE OIL, PARSLEY, CHAMOMILE, & HONEY

I will warn you; this procedure DOES work, but it IS work to make. (Wonder if that last drink was worth this?) Suck on a sugar cube containing a few drops of clove oil (a painkiller). Then chew on a sprig of parsley. Then drink a cup of lukewarm chamomile tea sweetened with honey. Then take a tsp. or two of plain honey, and repeat every ½ hr. for 2-3 hours. Parsley and chamomile both will calm an upset stomach.

HEADACHES

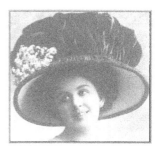

ALMONDS

Eat 10-12 almonds, the equivalent of two aspirins, for a migraine headache. Almonds are far less likely to upset the stomach.

ANISE SEED

"The perfume (scent) of anise seed taken up into the nose cureth headache."

APPLE

Apples are valuable in all types of headaches. After removing the upper rind and the inner hard portion of a ripe apple, it should be taken with a little salt every morning on an empty stomach in such cases. This should be continued for about a week.

BAKING SODA

A little soda water will relieve sick headache, caused by indigestion. Put about a tsp. or two of baking soda in a glass of water.

CINNAMON

Cinnamon is useful in headaches caused by exposure to cold air. A fine paste of this spice should be prepared by mixing it with water, and then it should be applied over the temples and forehead to obtain relief.

GARLIC

"The same (garlic) bruised betwixt the hands and laide to the temples, staketh the olde headache."

HANDKERCHIEF

Tie a kerchief or bandanna tightly around the head right above the eyebrows.

HONEY

Mix 3 large spoonfuls of honey in boiled water and drink. Honey has natural pain-relieving powers.

LEMON

There are several remedies for various types of headaches. Lemon is beneficial in its treatment. The juice of three or four slices of lemon should be squeezed in a cup of tea and taken by the patient for treating this condition. It gives immediate relief. The crust of lemon, which is generally thrown away, has been found useful in headaches caused by heat. Lemon crusts should be pounded into a fine paste in a mortar and applied as a plaster on the forehead. Applying the yellow, freshly pared-off rind of a lemon to each temple will also give relief.

ROSEMARY

For relieving tension headaches, infuse 1 tsp. dried rosemary tops, leaves, or flowers in 1 covered cup boiling water for 10 minutes. Strain and flavor with honey to taste. Drink while still warm as required. This tea is also effective as a stimulant and anti-depressive.

SAGE

To help relieve a nervous headache, infuse 1 tsp. dried leaves in 1 covered cup of boiling water. Strain after 10 minutes and sweeten with honey.

RED SAGE, CATNIP, PEPPERMINT OR SPEARMINT TEA

To relieve a nervous headache, take a cupful or two of any of these. Red sage is one of the best herbs for headache.

ROSEMARY

The herb rosemary has been found valuable in headaches resulting from cold. A handful of this herb should be boiled in a liter of water and put in a mug. The head should be covered with a towel and the steam inhaled for as long as the patient can bear. This should be repeated till the headache is relieved.

THYME

For headache, sore throat, coughs, and indigestion, infuse 1 tsp. dried thyme leaves in 1 c. boiling water for 10 minutes. Strain and flavor with honey. Drink as often as required.

VINEGAR

Soak compress with vinegar, chill it and apply to the forehead, temples, and neck. Even better, boil equal parts of vinegar and water and inhale the steam.

HEART DISEASE

ALFALFA

Mix about 1 tsp. - 1 Tbs. of fresh alfalfa juice into a glass of carrot juice and drink twice daily.

APPLE

Eat apples and drink apple juice liberally for heart-stimulating properties.

ASPARAGUS

Mix extracted juice from asparagus with honey in a ration of 2 to 1. Take 1 tsp. 3 times per day.

GRAPES

Grape juice is particularly valuable when one is or has suffered from a heart attack. It should be taken daily to control heart disease.

HONEY

Take 1 Tb. daily after every meal.

ONION

Take 1 tsp. of raw onion juice first thing each morning.

HEART PALPATATIONS

GRAPES

Grapes are one of the most effective home remedies for palpitation of the heart. The patient should take the juice of this fruit at frequent intervals. This will relieve the condition.

GUAVA The use of guava is another effective home remedy for palpitation of the heart The patient should eat a ripe guava daily on an empty stomach. It is especially beneficial if this disorder caused by nervousness and anemia.

HONEY

Honey has proved valuable in overcoming this condition. Honey is considered to be an excellent food for the heart, being easily digested and assimilated. The patient should take a glass of water, mixed with a tablespoon of honey and the juice of half a lemon before going to bed.

INDIAN SPIKENARD

The herb Indian spikenard is also beneficial in the treatment of palpitation of the heart It stimulates the action of the heart. It should be taken in doses of two to three grams with the addition of a pinch of camphor and cinnamon. It can also be taken as an infusion in doses of 30 to 60 ml, three times 1 a day.

HEMORRHOIDS

CASTOR OIL

When hemorrhoids come outside of the anal ring, castor oil will soften them so that they may be reversed.

GARLIC

Use a peeled, scraped clove of raw garlic as a suppository. The clove is left in place overnight and removed by normal bowel movements the following day. The process is repeated until the hemorrhoids disappear. Do not use if bleeding or tissue soreness is present.

GINGER

Mix ½ tsp. of fresh ginger juice with 1 tsp each of fresh lime juice, fresh mint juice and a Tbs. of honey and apply to affected area. Said to be an effective medicine for piles.

ONION

Apply raw, bruised onion to inflamed hemorrhoids. Do not use if bleeding or tissue soreness is present.

SORTING SCREWS

When I was 17, I was attending a junior college in Saratoga, California. My home had been in San Jose up to this point and this home had a swimming pool.

One afternoon I came home, full of excitement and expectation because Gukkie had flown in for one of her many visits from Chicago. As soon as I came in the door I asked my dad, "Where is she?" Chuckling, my father replied, "Out on the pool deck sorting screws." Sorting screws? This was a new one, even for her.

Gukkie could never just SIT. My mother is the same way. So am I. (Drives our husbands nuts.) Truly, we CAN sit but we have to be doing something while sitting. And Gukkie was the leader of the "do-something-while-sitting" pack.

Never one to be idle, Gukkie was always finding ways to make the best use of her time. There were always things to do and things to be done better. The funny part about her "doing" was that she was never "hyper" while doing. She had a free and easy-going attitude that nothing was impossible to tackle and never that hard. "Just be organized about it and it comes easy," was one of her many sayings.

When I went to the pool, Gukkie had just finished sorting thousands of screws, from minuscule to huge. When I asked her why she had done that she replied, "Well, when I was in the garage looking for a hammer on your dad's workbench (who knows what she was going to do with the hammer), I saw this box and thought he probably had a hard time finding a screw he needed for a certain project. They were all mixed up, so I sorted them. It was fun...like putting a puzzle together." Grief, I thought, Dad had told me it had taken her over two hours to sort those screws.

However, do you see what she did? She accomplished many things in one task (please, Lord, if my daughters read any of this book, let it be this story):

1. She saw a job that needed doing and didn't have to be asked to do it.

2. She wanted to help my father, so that he would have an easier time putting things together---because she loved him.

3. She didn't complain about the complexity or the time involved doing the task because…

4. She made it fun.

Why do we so often forget to add fun to our lives and take a brighter look at tasks before us? Why do we make even the smallest of chores seem so hard and lengthy? Most of us make life harder on ourselves than it is or needs to be.

Keep it simple. Gukkie sorted screws with joy throughout her life.

No matter how big or small the job, Gukkie was on it. And, she was smiling. Or humming. Or both.

HICCOUGHS: WHERE IS MARY POPPINS?

Nasty little buggers, hiccoughs are.

They always seem to time themselves out at the worst possible moments. And, you need that teaspoon of sugar or SOMETHING to get them to get lost.

Never fear, water is here.

I still use a favorite remedy of Gukkie's to get rid of hiccups. It sounds VERY weird but it works every time. (FYI: you look like a lunatic doing this, but what's worse? Hiccoughing during an important meeting or taking a second to drink water in a strange way - upside down?) Seriously.

Fill up a glass of water. Bend over and wrap your upper lip around the rim of the glass opposite you. Now drink the water. All of it (about a half of glass should do - 4 ounces). Now stand up. That's all, folks!

Gukkie said that when you have the hiccups, you have an air bubble "stuck down there" somewhere. When you drink the water upside down and then stand up, the water forces the air bubble to go "someplace else".

COLD WATER

"Take about a teacup full of cold water at nine sips, and the involuntary cough will cease."

DILL

Take 2 tsp. dried dill seeds. Bruise them in a pestle and mortar, and infuse them, covered, in 1/2 pint boiling water. Strain when cool, and take 2 oz. every hour or two until the condition is alleviated. This tea is also a digestive aid.

GINGER

Chew slices of fresh ginger slowly, swallowing the juice. You can also mix ginger juice with honey and drink slowly.

ORANGE

Cut an orange in half and drink the juice.

RICE VINEGAR

Mix rice vinegar with cold water and drink slowly.

SALT

Lick salt, letting it dissolve in your mouth, and then swallow it slowly.

INSECT BITES & RASHES

ALOE VERA PLANT

Treat insect bites by rubbing a slit lower leaf of an aloe vera plant onto the area.

AMMONIA

Strong ammonia dabbed onto a bee sting is most useful.

ASPIRIN

For an effective cure for a bee sting, rub the area with a moistened aspirin tablet.

BAKING SODA

Effective for bee stings: Mix baking soda and water into a paste and apply. This neutralizes most venom.

CORNSTARCH

Mix water with cornstarch into a paste and apply. This is effective in drawing out the poisons of most insect bites...and is also an effective remedy for diaper rash.

DIRT

For a wasp or bee sting, rub the area with damp earth. "The pain stops almost immediately and neither irritation of the skin nor swelling insects."

EPSOM SALTS & GLYCERIN

For a very effective mosquito repellent, fill half a tumbler with Epsom salts. Pour in just enough very hot water to melt it, add 20 drops of glycerin, and then rinse very lightly in the solution, two pieces of clean linen (about 9 inches square), and put them in a waterproof bag or old tobacco pouch. When in the open, pat all exposed flesh, especially well up on the back of the head and wrists, and let it dry on. Repeat if out long. It shows slightly on the face but is good for the complexion.

GARLIC

To ward off mosquitoes, rub garlic juice on exposed parts of body. Garlic is fatal to them.

HONEY

For a bee sting, remove the stinger, then coat the area with honey.

LEMON, VINEGAR, OR TEA

For wasp stings, one cannot beat using one of these weak acids.

MEAT TENDERIZER

To treat bee stings, sprinkle meat tenderizer on the area. Papaya is also a meat tenderizer and works as well, if not better, than those bought commercially..

OATMEAL

Add enough water to make a paste and apply to affected area. This helps to remedy itching and draw out the poison.

ONION

Put a slice of onion on a mosquito bite or bee sting.

POTATO

(Isn't there ANYTHING wrong with them?) For a wasp sting, rub it with slices of raw potato. If done at once, there will be hardly any swelling.

INSOMNIA

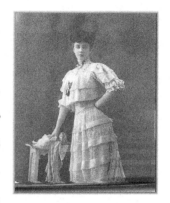

CALIFORNIA POPPY

California poppy is a member of the opium poppy family. It contains natural chemicals that have a sedative effect similar to that of codeine but it is much milder and not addictive. It is effective for nervous tension and anxiety that interfere with sleep. Pour one cup of boiling water over two teaspoons of dried herb, cover, and steep for 15 minutes. Strain, and sweeten if desired.

CURD

Curd is also useful in insomnia. The patient should take plenty of curd and massage it on the head. This will induce sleep.

HONEY

Honey is beneficial in the treatment of insomnia. It has a hypnotic action and induces a sound sleep. It should be taken with water before going to bed in doses of two teaspoons in a large cup of water.

HOPS

Hops is a potent sedative that has a relaxing effect on the central nervous system (it's one of the primary ingredients used in making beer). Hops is a good alternative for women who find that valerian causes agitation (see "Valerian"). However, if you are prone to depression, avoid using hops because it is a central nervous-system depressant. It can be difficult to find good-quality dried hops because the active ingredients break down quickly. Buy dried hops that are strongly aromatic and have a rich, golden-green color. Extracts tend to preserve more of the active ingredients. To make a tea, pour one cup of boiling water over one to two teaspoons of dried hops. Cover, and steep for 15 minutes. Strain, and sweeten if desired. Hops has a pleasantly bitter, rich flavor. As an alternative, take one-half teaspoon of the liquid extract in a small amount of warm water.

KAVA

Kava has a natural tranquilizing effect and is especially helpful for insomnia that is caused by anxiety. It contains compounds called kavalactones that are central nervous-system depressants and muscle relaxants. In small doses, kava acts to elevate mood, and in larger doses it acts as a sedative. Kava has a bitter, unpleasant flavor and is best used as an extract. Take one-half teaspoon of liquid extract or two capsules with warm water one hour before retiring. If you wish to take a standardized extract of kava, take enough capsules to provide 180 to 210 milligrams of kavalactones one hour before bed (approximately two to three capsules of an extract standardized for 60 to 75 milligrams of kavalactones per capsule).

LEMON BALM

Lemon Balm has been used for centuries as a mild tranquilizer, and in Germany it is a popular ingredient in herbal sedatives for insomnia. It has a light, lemony flavor and makes a mild sedative tea. Pour one cup of boiling water over two teaspoons of dried lemon balm. Cover, and steep for 15 minutes. Strain, and sweeten if desired.

LETTUCE

Lettuce is beneficial in the treatment of insomnia as it contains a sleep-inducing substance, called 'lectucarium'. The juice of this plant has been likened in effect to the sedative action of opium without the accompanying excitement. Lettuce seeds taken in a decoction are also useful in insomnia. One tablespoon of seeds should be boiled in half a liter of water, until it is reduced by one-third and taken by tablespoon as needed.

MILK

Milk is very valuable in insomnia. A glass of milk, sweetened with honey, should be taken every night before going to bed in treating this condition. It acts as a tonic and a tranquilizer. Massaging the milk over the soles of the feet has also been found effective.

PASSION FLOWER

Passion Flower has been used for centuries by Native Americans and Europeans as a sleep aid and is included in many sleep preparations in Britain and Germany. It has mild tranquilizing and sedative properties and promotes restful sleep. To make a pleasant-tasting tea, pour one cup of water over two teaspoons of dried herb, cover, and steep for 15 minutes. Strain, and sweeten if desired.

ST. JOHN'S WORT

St. John's Wort can be helpful for relieving chronic insomnia that is caused by anxiety or depression. St. John's Wort does not provide immediate relief---it usually takes a couple of months of consistent use to begin to feel the effects. If you want to try St. John's Wort, take an extract standardized to contain 0.3 percent hypericin, 300 milligrams three times a day. The following herbs are some of the most helpful for treating insomnia.

THIAMINE

Of the various food elements, thiamine or vitamin B1 is of special significance in the treatment of insomnia. It is vital for strong, healthy nerves. A body starved of thiamine over a long period will be unable to relax and fall asleep naturally. Valuable sources of this vitamin are wholegrain cereals, pulses, and nuts.

VALERIAN

Valerian has been used for hundreds of years in China, India, and Europe to treat insomnia and is excellent as a non-addictive sleep aid. It calms the nervous system and helps to quickly induce sleep. For a small percentage of women, valerian causes agitation instead of relaxation. If you've never used valerian before it's best to begin with a small dose and then to increase the amount if you have positive results. If you find it to be stimulating, try hops or kava instead. Because valerian has a very pungent odor and flavor, most women find it easier to take it as an extract or in capsules. To use valerian as a sedative for sleep, you need to use a larger amount than if you are using it to simply relieve anxiety. Take one to two teaspoons of valerian extract or two to three capsules with a small amount of warm water 30 minutes before bed. If necessary, repeat the dose after 30 minutes.

LEG & FOOT PROBLEMS

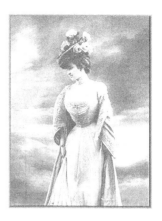

ALOE VERA GEL, CORNSTARCH, WITCH HAZEL & PEPPERMINT OIL

Combine 1/2 c. aloe vera gel, 1 1/2 tsp. cornstarch, and 1 Tb. witch hazel into a heat-resistant container. Warm the mixture until you have a clear, thick liquid, about the consistency of honey. After the mixture has cooled, add 3-4 drops peppermint oil and stir thoroughly. Pour into an airtight container. Massage into legs and feet - a wonderful treat for someone with leg and foot problems, as well as a great "pick me up" for someone who doesn't.

BLACKSTRAP MOLASSES

For varicose veins, take 2-3 tsp. of blackstrap molasses daily. This also treats all kinds of circulatory ailments.

CIDER VINEGAR

To treat varicose veins, massage legs with the vinegar to shrink the veins and to relieve the related cramping and muscle tiredness. Another method is to soak bandages in cider vinegar and wrap around unsightly veins. Lie down, elevate your legs, and relax for at least an hour or more. Do this twice a day. And follow each session by drinking 2 tsp. of the vinegar in a cup of warm water. You should notice a difference within a month.

HONEY

Eat honey to curb leg and foot pain. Honey is a natural painkiller.

MENOPAUSE

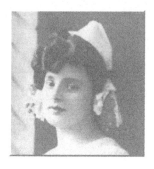

BLACK COHOSH

Touted as one of the best treatments by physicians for menopausal symptoms, black cohosh has estrogen-like properties that treat hot flashes, vaginal dryness, and depression. Take as directed.

GINGER

Pound a piece of fresh ginger and boil in 1 c. of water for about 3 minutes. Sweeten with sugar. "Take thrice daily after meals for menstrual disorders."

PARSLEY

Mix equal parts of parsley juice with beet, carrot, or cucumber juice. Take daily to regulate cycles.

SESAME SEEDS

"Half a teaspoon of the powder of these seeds, taken with hot water twice daily, acts excellently in reducing spasmodic pain (cramps) during menstruation in young, unmarried girls."

TEA BLEND FOR CRAMPS

3 tsp. freshly grated ginger root

3 tsp. chamomile

2 c. water

Simmer ginger root and water in a covered pt for 10 minutes. Remove from heat and add chamomile. Cover and steep for 10 minutes. Strain, sweeten with sugar or honey if desired and drink as needed.

PSORIASIS

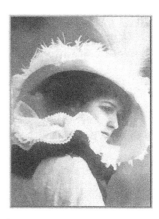

AVOCADO OIL

The oil of avocado has been found beneficial in the treatment of this disease. It should be applied gently to the affected parts.

BITTER GOURD

Bitter gourd is a valuable remedy for psoriasis. A cup of fresh juice of this vegetable, mixed with a teaspoon of lime juice, should be taken sip by sip, on an empty stomach daily for four to six months.

BUTTERMILK

The use of curd in the form of buttermilk has proved useful in psoriasis and the patient should drink it in liberal quantities. The application of buttermilk compresses over the affected parts will also be useful in treating this condition.

CABBAGE LEAVES

Cabbage leaves have been successfully used in the form of compresses in the treatment of psoriasis. The thickest and greenest outer leaves are most effective for use as compresses. They should be thoroughly washed in warm water and dried with a towel. The leaves should be flattened, softened and smoothed out by rolling them with a rolling pin after removing the thick veins. They should be warmed and then applied smoothly to the affected part in an overlapping manner. A pad of soft "woollen" cloth should be put over them. The whole compress should then be secured with an elastic bandage.

CASHEW NUT OIL

The oil extracted from the outer shell of the cashew nut is acrid, and then applied beneficially on the affected area.

LECITHIN

Lecithin is also considered a remarkable remedy for psoriasis. The patient may take six to nine lecithin capsules a day—two or three capsules before or after each meal. If taken in the form of granules, four tablespoonfuls may be taken daily for two months. The dosage may be reduced thereafter to two tablespoons.

VITAMIN E

Vitamin E therapy has been found effective in the treatment of psoriasis. The patient should take this vitamin in therapeutic doses of 400 mg a day. It will help reduce itching and scab formation.

STOMACHACHES, INDIGESTION, ULCERS, & NAUSEA

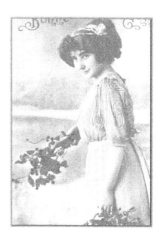

ALMONDS

Milk prepared from blanched almonds in a blender is very useful as a treatment for peptic ulcers. It binds the excess of acid in the stomach and supplies high quality protein.

ANISE SEED

A very effective remedy for indigestion is to chew on anise seeds or drink as a strong tea: 1 tsp. seed to 1 c. water. Cover and steep 10-15 minutes. This remedy is also effective to babies with colic.

APPLE CIDER VINEGAR CURE

For diarrhea and vomiting put 1 tsp. vinegar in a glass of water. Give 1 tsp. of mixture every 5 minutes. When there is food poisoning with vomiting, you should attempt to drink the whole glass at once.

BASIL

Infuse 1 tsp. dried basil in 1 covered cup of boiling water, strain, and flavor with honey, if desired. Up to 1-2 cups per day can be taken for mild, nervous tension headaches or nausea.

BANANA

Banana is one of the most effective home remedies for the treatment of a peptic ulcer. This fruit is said to contain an unidentified compound, perhaps jokingly called vitamin U (against ulcers). Banana neutralizes the over-acidity of the gastric juices and reduces the irritation of the ulcer by coating the lining of the stomach. Patients who are in an advanced state of the disease should take a diet consisting only of two bananas with a glass of milk, three or four times a day.

BUTTERMILK

A very simple remedy for indigestion is a glass of thin buttermilk mixed with a quarter teaspoon of pepper powder. For better results an equal quantity of cumin powder may be added to the buttermilk.

CABBAGE

Cabbage is regarded as another useful home remedy for a peptic ulcer: 250 gm should be boiled in 500 ml water till it is reduced to half; this water should be allowed to cool, and taken twice daily. The juice extracted from raw cabbage is also a valuable medicine for a peptic ulcer. However, as this juice is very strong, it should be taken in combination with carrot juice, in quantities of 125 ml each.

CARROT

Carrots are valuable in treating indigestion. The chewing of this vegetable increases saliva and quickens digestion by supplying the necessary enzymes, minerals, and vitamins. Half a glass of carrot juice, diluted with an equal quantity of water, can be taken once daily to treat this disorder.

CATNIP

Warm catnip tea, given in a bottle, will treat the symptoms of colic; indigestion, improper food and constipation.

CAYENNE PEPPER

Take as much cayenne pepper as you can rightly bear in a bowl of hot soup, and the nausea (including from seasickness) will disappear.

CHAMOMILE TEA

Chamomile tea is said to be far more relaxing than most stomach remedies. Buy the commercial type or steep 1 tsp. chamomile flowers in 1 c. of water (covered) for 10 minutes. Add honey if desired.

CHAMOMILE WINE

To settle the stomach, add 1 handful of chamomile flowers to 1 bottle white wine or Madeira red wine. Steep for up to 10 days. Strain. Use in Tb. doses.

CINNAMON

A simple cure for a stomachache is to dissolve 4g of ground cinnamon in 1 c. of warm water, cover it for 15 minutes, and drink it like tea. This remedy can also ease diarrhea and flatulence.

CINNAMON BARK & CARDAMOM SEED

For nausea, grind 3 small cinnamon sticks or one 6-inch stick with 1 Tb. (about 8 seeds) of cardamom. Use a nut grinder, coffee grinder, or blender. Place the mixture in a labeled jar and use 1/4 tsp. in 1 c. hot tea for relief. Use a tiny pinch of the powder for a child.

COCONUT

Coconut water is an excellent remedy for gastritis. It gives the stomach the necessary rest and provides vitamins and minerals. The stomach is greatly helped in returning to a normal condition if nothing but coconut water is given during the first 24 hours.

FENUGREEK SEEDS

A tea made from fenugreek seeds is yet another useful remedy for peptic ulcers. The seeds, when moistened with water, are slightly mucilaginous. The tea helps in the healing of ulcers as the mild coating of mucilaginous material deposited by fenugreek, passes through the stomach and intestines, providing protective shell for the ulcers.

GINGER

For nausea, make ginger tea by mixing 1/2 tsp. dried ginger in a cup of tea. Ginger root, grated, and made into a tea also relieves motion sickness.

GOAT'S MILK

Goat's milk is also highly beneficial in the treatment of this disease. It actually helps to heal peptic ulcers. For better results, a glass of goat's milk should be taken in a raw state, three times daily.

GRAPES

The use of grapes is another effective remedy for indigestion. This fruit is a light food and removes indigestion and irritation of the stomach in a short time. About 250 gm can be taken daily.

HONEY

Honey is a digestive aid used to prevent heartburn and gas. Take 1 tsp. before and after meals as needed. Honey also soothes irritated ulcers.

RED CLOVER

Red clover tea (obtained at health food stores) is very effective in cleansing the system. Use the blossoms, one tsp. to a cup of boiling water. Steep, and drink from 5-12 cups a day.

LEMON

The use of fruits in general is beneficial in the treatment of indigestion. They flush out the undigested food residue and accumulated feces, and re-establish health to perfect order. The best fruit for die treatment of indigestion is lemon. Its juice reaches the stomach and attacks the bacteria, inhibiting the formation of acids.

Lemon juice removes indigestion by dislodging this acid and other harmful substances from the stomach, thereby strengthening and promoting a healthy appetite. The juice of one lemon, diluted with water, can be taken twice daily before each main meal.

LEMON & HONEY

A morning tonic is made by mixing 2 Tb. lemon juice with 2 Tb. of honey in an ounce of water. Relieves flatulence.

LIME

Lime is valuable in peptic ulcers. The citric acid in this fruit, together with the mineral salts present in the juice, help in digestion.

MARIGOLD

The herb marigold is also considered beneficial in the treatment of gastritis. An infusion of the herb in doses of a tablespoon may be taken twice daily.

MARJORAM

Excellent for any type of upset stomach: Infuse 1 tsp. dried leaves in 1 covered cup boiling water for 15 minutes. Strain and flavor with honey, if desired. Up to 2 cups per day may be taken.

MINT

Mint is also very useful in correcting indigestion because of its digestive properties. Mint juice is a good appetizer. One teaspoon of mint juice, mixed with an equal amount of honey and lemon juice, forms a very effective remedy for indigestion and gaseous distension of the stomach.

MINT LEAVES

Put two mint leaves in a steaming cup of tea to make a relaxing and effective indigestion remedy.

MUSTARD

Dissolve 1 tsp. ground mustard in 1 c. warm water to relieve heartburn. This remedy is also good for hiccoughs.

OREGANO

An age-old recipe for use as a digestive aid and to expel worms: Use 1-2 tsp. of dried herb per cup of boiling water. Steep 10 minutes. Drink up to 3 cups per day.

PINEAPPLE OR PMEGRANATE JUICE

Another fruit useful in indigestion is pineapple. It acts as a tonic and relieves much of the digestive disorders of the dyspeptics. Half a glass of pineapple juice should be taken after one meal in treating this condition. Pomegranate: One tablespoon of pomegranate juice, mixed with a tablespoon of honey, is valuable in indigestion accompanied by giddiness. This dose may be taken twice daily. The seeds of this fruit act as a stomach tonic when mixed with a little rock salt and Mack pepper powder.

POTATO

Potato juice has been found valuable in relieving gastritis. The recommended dose is half a cup of the juice, two or three times daily, half an hour before meals.

RICE: Rice gruel is another excellent remedy for acute cases of gastritis. One cup of rice gruel is recommended twice daily. In chronic cases where the flow of gastric juice is meagre, such foods as require prolonged vigorous mastication are beneficial as they induce a greater flow of gastric juice.

VEGETABLE JUICES

The juices of raw vegetables, particularly carrot and cabbage, are beneficial in the treatment of peptic ulcers. Carrot juice may be taken either alone or in combination with spinach, or beet and cucumber. The formula proportions in case of the first combination are 300 ml of carrot juice and 200 ml of spinach juice; and in case of the second combination, 300 ml of carrot juice and 100 ml each of beet and cucumber juice to make 500 ml of juice.

WOOD APPLE

An infusion of the leaves of wood apple is another effective remedy for this disease. 15 grams of leaves should be soaked overnight in 250 ml of water. In the morning this water should be strained and taken as a drink. The pain and discomfort will be relieved when this treatment is continued for a few weeks. Bael leaves are rich in tannins which reduce inflammation and help in the healing of ulcers. The bad fruit taken in the form of a beverage also has great healing properties on account of its mucilage content. This substance forms a coating on the stomach mucosa and thus helps in the healing of ulcers.

CHURCH

There's a chair in a quiet part of the room by a window where you can see the golden colors of the new dawn. The birds are getting up and singing their morning songs. The grass is green and the world is quiet except for the serene sounds around you. The sun is coming up yet another day, and you are thanking something or someone, that you have enough of a purpose on this planet to experience it all.

One time when I was about 14 years old, I saw Gukkie, as I had so many times before, in this atmosphere. "Up with the birds," my dad used to say about her. She always kept this time, every day, as her time to meditate, to pray, and to be thankful.

When I asked Gukkie why she didn't go to church when she visited us, she just smiled. I had caught her during one these tranquil mornings, and she not only smiled---she glowed.

Gukkie responded to my question, smiling with dimples highlighted. She said, "Church is in your heart, not in a building. I carry my church with me wherever I go. Because I love the Lord and I know He loves me. and I'm so glad to be here today to talk to you...and your mother, and sister, and your dad. I'm thankful for all that I have and am, and that's why I have a joyous heart."

Gukkie taught me a very valuable lesson that one morning. I still treasure my mornings, even if they're afternoons, for even a small block of time I can grab for myself, to do exactly what she did. The bathtub seems to be my own favorite spot. Whatever time I can take to "break away" to regroup, I hop in the tub. It makes an enormous difference to the outcome of your day.

I'm always counting my own blessings during these periods, taking stock of what I have in my life---not what I don't have (yet).

You are special enough to be counted among many other people, to fulfill some purpose in life. A very special purpose that you may not be aware of right now. Be thankful that you have opportunities to make YOUR mark. Gukkie IMPRINTED hers on scores of hearts and souls.

When Gukkie had the opportunity to attend church, she may not have sang the loudest. However she would be the first one with a tear of joy rolling down her cheek, and her face upturned toward the sun, not downwardward.

And, her hands would be clasped as if holding something precious.

STRESS & DEPRESSION

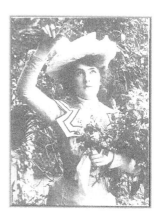

APPLE

Apple is one of the most valuable remedies for mental depression. The various chemical substances present in this fruit such as vitamin B, phosphorus, and potassium help the synthesis of glutamic acid, which controls the wear and tear of nerve cells. The fruit should be taken with milk and honey. This remedy will act as a very effective nerve tonic and recharge the nerves with new energy and life.

APPLE CIDER VINEGAR & HONEY

To overcome chronic fatigue and depression, use 1 tsp. of each to a glass of water. Additionally for insomnia, you can add 3 Tbs. of vinegar to 1 c. of honey. Take 2 tsp. of the mixture on preparing for bed.

ASPARAGUS

The root of asparagus has been found beneficial in the treatment of depression. It is highly nutritious and is used as an herbal medicine for mental disorders. It is a good tonic for the brain and nerves. One or two grams of the powder of the dry root of the plant can be taken once daily.

BORAGE & WINE

As an antidepressant, make a drink consisting of 2 Tb. borage in 1 liter of dark or light wine. Seal, and put in a dark, cool place for 10 days. Strain and take by the teaspoonful as needed.

CARDAMOM

The use of cardamom has proved valuable in depression. Powdered seeds should be boiled in water and tea prepared in the usual way. Cardamom has a very pleasing aroma when added to the tea and very effective in the treatment of this condition.

CASHEW NUT

The cashew nut is another valuable remedy for general depression and nervous weakness. It is rich in vitamins of die B group, especially thiamine and is therefore useful in stimulating the appetite and the nervous system. It is also rich in riboflavin which keeps the body active, cheerful, and energetic.

COFFEE

To help get rid of mild depression, drink 1 c. of coffee (no more than 2) per day.

HONEY & WATER

Energizing Mead recipe: Simmer 1 c. honey and 3 c. water together slowly. Allow one c. of the water to evaporate. Strain off the top surface, and put the remaining liquid into a stoneware crock or dark bottle. Put a towel over it so it can breathe, yet be free of dirt. Place in a cool place. You can add cinnamon, clove, or the juice of 2 lemons, if you like. Sip as needed.

ROSE

An infusion of rose petals should be prepared by mixing 15 gm of rose petals in 250 ml of boiling water. If drunk occasionally, instead of the usual tea and coffee, it is beneficial for treating this condition.

SPINACH

3/4 c. of cooked spinach a day is enough to give dramatic relief from depression if you are deficient in B vitamins

VITAMIN B

Diet has a profound effect on the mental health of a person. Even a single nutritional deficiency can cause depression in susceptible people. Nutritional therapy builds up brain chemicals, such as serotonin and nor epinephrine, that affect the mood and are often lacking in depressed people. Eating foods rich in vitamin B, such as whole grains, green vegetables, eggs, and fish helps restore vitality and cheer in an individual.

THROAT AILMENTS

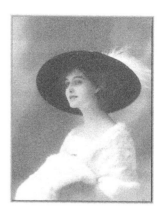

ANISE SEED, HONEY, & COGNAC

Boil 1/2 c. of anise seeds in 1 c. of water for 50 minutes. Stain, then stir in 1/4 honey and 1 Tb. cognac. Take 1 Tb. every 30 minutes. as systems persist.

ANISE TEA

Anise mint tea is very good for sore throats. Use 1 teaspoon dried anise mint for each cup of boiling water. Let steep 10 minutes. Strain and sweeten. Drink as warm as possible. Repeat as often as desired.

APPLE CIDER VINEGAR

Apply an apple cider compress to the throat, bind it with a large wool, and then bind it with a larger wool compress on top of that. This relieves even the most painful sore throat.

BACON & PEPPER

"Hardly any remedy for sore throat proves more efficacious than the old fashioned plan of tying around the throat a slice of bacon on which is laid black pepper."

BLACK CURRENT LEAVES

Place 2 tablespoons of chopped black currant leaves in 1 cup of water. Simmer for 15 minutes. Strain and cool. Use as a gargle to relieve a sore throat.

BORAGE

Make a tea using 1/2cup of borage leaves to 2 cups of boiling water. Steep for 30 minutes. Strain and refrigerate. Use as a gargle when needed for sore throats.

BRANDY

Add 1/2 cup of brown sugar to 1/2 cup of brandy. Mix well and sip as needed to relieve a sore throat.

CAYENNE

Mix 1 teaspoon cayenne pepper with 1 cup boiling water. Drink 3 times daily to stop or ward off colds and sore throats. This does work very well. The length of the illness is drastically reduced.

CINNAMON

Cinnamon is regarded as an effective remedy for a sore throat resulting from a cold. One teaspoon of coarser/ powdered cinnamon, boiled in a glass of water with a pinch of pepper powder, and two teaspoons of honey can be taken as a medicine in the treatment of this condition. Two or three drops of cinnamon oil, mixed with a teaspoon of honey, also gives immense relief.

FENUGREEK SEEDS

A gargle prepared from fenugreek seeds has been found to be a very effective remedy for dealing with a sore throat. To prepare this gargle, two tablespoons of fenugreek seeds should be put in a liter of cold water and allowed to 1/2 an hour over a low flame. This should then be allowed to cool to a bearable temperature, strained, and then used entirely as a gargle.

GINGER, LEMON, & HONEY

Pour 1/2 c. boiling water over 1 tsp. powdered ginger. Add 1/2 c. squeezed lemon and 1 tsp. honey. Gargle.

GRAPEFRUIT

Squeeze the juice from a grapefruit, gargle it, and drink whatever is left over.

HONEY

Take a tsp. of honey, place it on your tongue, and let it trickle down your throat.

HORSERADISH, HONEY, & GROUND CLOVES

Add 1 Tb. grated fresh horseradish (dried is not as effective), 1 tsp. honey, and 1 tsp. ground cloves to a glass of warm water. Stir and sip slowly, or use as a gargle. Do not take large amounts. Discontinue if diarrhea occurs.

MANGO BARK

Mango bark is efficacious in the treatment of a sore throat and other throat disorders. Its fluid, which is extracted by grinding, can be applied locally with beneficial results. It can also be used as a throat gargle. This gargle is prepared by mixing 10 ml of the fluid extract with 125 ml of water.

MARJORAM

To relieve sore throat pain, dip a cotton cloth into a strong marjoram tea 1-2 tsp. marjoram to 1 c. covered boiling water), and wrap around the throat. Overwrap with a larger, warm flannel cloth. Make sure it is as airtight as possible.

POMEGRANATE

Dry a pomegranate rind. Add 2 tablespoons of the dried and grated pomegranate rind to 2 cups of water. Bring to a boil and reduce heat. Simmer the mixture until it is reduced by half. Strain and add 1/4 cup of sugar. Gargle with the liquid as needed.

SAGE

Pour 2 cups of boiling water over 2 tablespoons of dried sage and 1/2 teaspoon of cayenne pepper. Steep overnight and use as a gargle.

SAGE & LARD

This old recipe is intended to protect and keep medicinal properties of sage in the throat as long as possible: Simmer a handful of sage in enough lard to cover herb. When most of the properties of the herb are extracted, strain off, and repeat process with a fresh batch of sage. Strain off herb. When sufficiently cool, give in 1 tsp. doses three or four times a day as needed.

SHERRY, CLOVE, CINNAMON & CARAWAY

Strain 2 Tbs. bruised cloves, 1 Tb. bruised cinnamon, and a pinch of bruised caraway seed in 1 pint inexpensive sherry. After a week or two, strain out herbs. For one more week, keep the mixture in a dark closet, shaking as often as you can. Add about 1 tsp. to a glass of water and gargle as needed.

SLIPPERY ELM

Make a paste using 1 tablespoon slippery elm powder, and just enough water to make a paste. Dissolve 1/2 cup of honey in 2 cups of boiling water. Add honey water slowly to slippery elm paste. Take 1 tablespoon as needed.

TAMARIND

Tamarind is also beneficial in the treatment of this condition. Tamarind water should be used as a gargle. A powder of the dry leaves and an infusion of the bark can also be used for preparation of a gargle for treating sore throat.

VINEGAR

Mix 2 cups vinegar with 1 cup of honey. Drink a wineglass of this mixture 3 times daily.

USE THIS AT THE FIRST SIGN OF A SORE THROAT

Mix 2 tablespoons honey; 1/2 teaspoon cayenne pepper, 4 tablespoons apple cider vinegar, and 1 tablespoon of lemon juice to 1 cup warm water. Mix well and use as a gargle.

TOOTH & MOUTH PROBLEMS

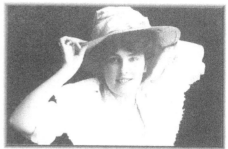

CLOVE

Bruised leaves of clove can be placed in the mouth on the affected tooth. Oil of cloves, a strong antiseptic, can be used on a plug of cotton to pack a cavity until you can get to a dentist.

CLOVE #2

The use of a clove in toothache reduces pain. It also helps to decrease infection due to its antiseptic properties. Clove oil, applied to a cavity in a decayed tooth, also relieves toothache.

DRIED FIG & MILK

Cook a dried fig in milk and apply it to the painful area.

GARLIC

Chew on a clove of garlic, or hold it against the tooth. The antibacterial properties of garlic are well-known. Another recipe is : "pounde with vinegar, and laid to the teeth."

GARLIC #2

Garlic is one of most effective of several home remedies for toothache. A clove of garlic with a little rock salt should be placed on the affected tooth. It will relieve the pain and, sometimes, may even cure it. A clove should also be chewed daily in the morning. It will make the teeth strong and healthy.

GUAVA

Chewing unripe guava is an excellent tonic for the teeth and gums. It stops the bleeding from the gums due to its styptic effect and richness in vitamin C. Chewing the tender leaves of the guava tree also helps in curing bleeding from the gums and keeps the teeth healthy. A decoction of root-bark can also be beneficially used as a mouthwash for swollen gums.

LEMON & LIME

The regular use of lemon and lime is useful in pyorrhea due to their high vitamin C content. They strengthen the gums and teeth and are very effective in preventing and curing acute inflammations of the gum.

LIME

Lime, as a rich source of vitamin C, is useful in maintaining the health of the teeth and other bones of the body. It prevents decay and loosening of the teeth, dental cavaties, toothache and bleeding of gums.

LETTUCE

Lettuce has proved useful in preventing pyorrhea. The leaves of this vegetable should be chewed every day, immediately after meals for this purpose.

ONION

Latest research has confirmed the bactericidal properties of onion. If a person consumes one raw onion every day by thorough mastication, he will be protected from a host of disorders. Chewing raw onion for three minutes is sufficient to kill all the germs in the mouth. Toothache is often allayed by placing a small piece of onion on the bad tooth or gum.

ORANGE

The use of orange has also been found beneficial in the treatment of pyorrhea. This fruit should be eaten regularly and its skin rubbed over the teeth and gums. This will improve the condition.

PEPPER

A mixture of a pinch of pepper powder and a quarter teaspoon of common salt is an excellent dentifrice. Its daily use prevents dental caries, foul breath, bleeding from the gums, painful gums, and toothaches. It cures the increased sensitiveness of the teeth. A pinch of pepper powder mixed with clove oil can be put on cavities to alleviate the toothache.

PEPPERMINT & SALT

To ease toothache or other mouth pain, make a tea by boiling 5g of fresh peppermint in 1 C. water and adding a little salt. Peppermint is an antiseptic and contains menthol, which relieves pain when applied to skin surfaces.

POMEGRANATE RIND

Powder of the dry rind of pomegranate, mixed with pepper and common salt, can be applied as a very good dentifrice. Its regular application strengthens the gums, stops bleeding, and prevents pyorrhea.

SALT

For an antiseptic mouthwash and gargle, combine 1 tsp. salt in 1 c. warm water. Dissolve salt. Works best when warm.

SALT AND ALUM

Mix 1/2 teaspoon each of salt and alum. Pack in and around the tooth for quick pain relief.

SPINACH JUICE

The juice of raw spinach is another valuable remedy for the prevention and treatment of pyorrhea because of its beneficial effect on the teeth and gums. This effect is greatly enhanced if spinach juice is taken in combination with carrot juice. Both spinach juice and carrot juice should be taken in quantities of 125 ml each daily. A permanent aid for this affliction has been found in the use of natural raw foods, and in drinking an ample quantity of carrot and spinach juice.

STRAWBERRY

Cut a strawberry in half, then each half is rubbed over the teeth and gums. Strawberries whiten teeth and remove plaque, as well.

STRAWBERRY LEAVES & LEMON

For an effective and antiseptic mouthwash, take 1/4 c. dried or 1 c. fresh strawberry leaves and pour 1 c. boiling water over them. Cool and strain off the liquid. Add 2 tsp. lemon juice to the liquid and stir well. Store in refrigerator. To use, pour 4 tsp. in a glass and rinse mouth for 30 seconds.

VANILLA

Put several drops of vanilla extract directly on the affected tooth to stop the ache.

VODKA, HONEY, CINNAMON, & GROUND CLOVES OR CLOVE OIL

For a clove mouthwash, combine 1/4 c. vodka, 1/2 c distilled water, 1/4 tsp. honey, 1/4 tsp. cinnamon, and 1/2 tsp. clove and stir well until the honey is dissolved. Filter if ground cloves were used. To use, pour about 4 tsp. into a glass and rinse mouth for 30 seconds.

TOOTH POWDERS & MOUTH WASHES

ANISE SEEDS

For fresh breath, chew on anise seeds.

BAKING SODA

Dip a damp toothbrush into the box and use to brush teeth instead of toothpaste. Baking soda has just the right consistency for a dentifrice, and has enough scouring action to remove plaque.

BORAX

A good pinch in 1/2 glass of warm water makes a good wash for the mouth and teeth, or the powder can be sprinkled on the toothbrush and used in the usual way.

CARDAMOM SEEDS

Chew on cardamom seeds to cleanse and sweeten breath. Cardamom seeds also cover up alcohol on the breath.

CLOVES

Chew on 1 or 2 cloves to get rid of bad breath.

CLOVES, CINNAMON, HONEY, VODKA & WATER

Take 1/2 c. water, 1/4 c. vodka, 1/4 tsp. honey, 1/4 tsp. cinnamon, and 1/2 tsp. ground cloves or clove oil and combine. Stir well until the honey is dissolved. Pour into a clean bottle. Filter first if you have used ground cloves. To use, pour about 4 tsp. into a glass and rinse mouth for 30 seconds. Makes 5 oz.

HYDROGEN PEROXIDE

Hydrogen peroxide has an effervescence that can float away particles from between your teeth and has bacteriostatic properties. A highly effective method of maintain dental hygiene is to first soak your toothbrush in hydrogen peroxide, and then dip it in baking soda before brushing.

PARSLEY

Chewing on a sprig of parsley can eliminate garlic and alcohol breath.

PARSLEY, MINT, & VODKA

For an herbal mouthwash, combine 2 Tb. fresh parsley, 2 Tb. fresh mint, 1 c. distilled water, and 1 Tb. vodka in a blender. Blend well for 2 minutes, strain, and pour into a container. To use, pour about 4 tsp. in a glass and rinse mouth for 30 seconds.

PEPPERMINT, THYME LEAVES, CLOVES, NUTMEG, PEPPERMINT OIL & SHERRY

For a mint mouthwash combine 1/2 tsp. dried peppermint, 1/2 tsp. dried thyme leaves, 1/2 tsp. crushed cloves, 1/2 tsp. freshly grated nutmeg, and 1/2 pint sherry or white wine. Steep herbs in sherry or wine only for a week to 10 days. Strain out the herbs, add 10 drops of peppermint oil, and label.

SAGE, BAKING SODA, & SALT

For a tooth-whitening powder, mix 1 tsp. of each and dip damp toothbrush into mixture. Brush for 2 minutes.

WARTS, CALLUSES, & CORNS

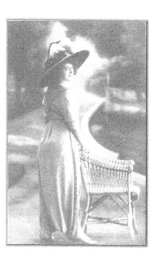

BAKING SODA

Soaking the feet in baking soda and water will also dissolve the corn.

CASTOR OIL

Rub a mixture of castor oil and finely grated raw garlic on a corn to remove it.

CHALK POWDER

Chalk powder has also been found beneficial in the treatment of corns. A small piece of chalk may be ground into a paste with water and applied over the affected area.

GARLIC

Try taping a slice of garlic to the wart. Be sure to first protect the surrounding skin with petroleum jelly. You can also pulverize garlic and bind over the corn and leave on overnight.

IVY LEAVES

Soak bruised ivy leaves in vinegar overnight. Soak a small piece of bread in the vinegar mixture and apply to corn. Bind and leave on during the day. Refresh with fresh application at night. Continue treatment until corn is gone.

LEMON

Bind a slice of lemon to the corn or callus and leave on overnight, and each night thereafter until the corn or callus disappears.

LICORICE

Grind three or four black licorice sticks with ½ tsp. sesame or mustard oil to make a thick paste. Rub into corn before bedtime to soften and reduce its size.

ONION

Place a slice of raw onion over the corn every night and bind. Said to remove corns in 3-4 weeks.

PINEAPPLE

If a thin slice of pineapple be kept in close contact with a corn for 8 hours, the corn will become so soft as to admit easy removal.

PAPAYA

Raw papaya is beneficial in the treatment of corns. Its juice is an irritant and it is, therefore; a useful application in this condition. Half a teaspoon of raw papaya juice may be applied thrice daily.

POTATO

To remove warts, rub the white part of a raw potato on the wart. According to folklore, the piece of potato was buried after use, or the cure was not effective.

ROCKING CHAIR

I know the movie exists even though I haven't seen it in a long time. It's on 8mm film and recorded during the days when that was all there was.

The last time I saw this film was during yet another Christmas, except this time, WE were in Illinois. I was at my great uncle's house one evening during this visit and the whole family had gathered around to watch our legendary family and our antics. (I could tell you some stories about my mother but I don't think she'd find it funny being even remotely compared to "I Love Lucy" - hey, mom, remember the frog that came up the drain in the shower at the cabin...while you were in it?....)

Anyway, this one particular film impressed me, not so much because of its hilarity, but because I caught a message.

In this film, my great-aunt (great-uncle's first wife) who was suffering and dying from cancer, was sitting in a rocking chair during a previous holiday evening. (She had since passed away by the time we saw this film.) Gukkie, who was her caregiver at the time, was somewhere nearby.

The aunt gets up, and the next shot is of Gukkie in the rocking chair, rocking away like the thing is going to sprout wings and take off. The next frames are of the rocking chair rocking with no one sitting in it.

Everyone laughed at the time, how funny that looked, the rocking chair going back and forth like crazy with no one in it. And, I thought it was funny, too, at first. But then I thought about how unbelievable that would look to someone who didn't see the first part of the film showing the women who sat in the chair to begin with and had propelled the rocker's motions.

The rocking chair "rocked on" in that film shot so many years ago.

In addition, do you know what? It still does, thanks to the women who started its motions.

I know this because I'm living proof. And these women have made me very proud to be a part of a pretty incredible family of "Motherhood and Sisterhood" and for teaching me to be the best I can be no matter what life brings.

Again, to Gukkie and all the many other women who have gone before me to lay a blueprint to make my own life's journey easier to follow I say,

"Thank You."

OLD-TIME HOUSEHOLD TIPS & HINTS

To Remove Tar

From hands or clothing, rub well with lard then wash well with soap and water.

To Keep Ants Away

To keep ants away from any dish or pail, draw a circle of chalk around it.

To Take Out Scorch

Lay the article out where the bright sunlight will fall directly on it. It will take the scorch entirely out.

To Make Sour Fruit Sweet Without Sugar

To two pounds of fruit when cooking, add one tsp. of baking soda.

To Give Gloss To House Plants

Dip a bit of cotton in milk and dab and wipe leaves carefully.

If A Fountain Pen Gets Clogged

Fill pen with vinegar to clean it.

To Remove Water Stains

Dampen the entire material evenly and then press while damp.

To Remove Fruit Stains

From white or colorfast material, stretch material over a bowl and pour boiling water through it from a height of about three feet. Soap will ALWAYS SET fruit stains.

To Remove Iron Rust From White Goods

Rub out with milk.

To Remove Rust

Use lemon juice and salt.

To Remove Vegetable Stains From Hands

Rub hands with raw potato.

To Remove Dried Mud & Soil Spots From Clothing

Rub a raw potato on the spots.

To Remove Fresh Ink Stains

Place material immediately in sweet milk. Or dip the garment in apple cider vinegar and rub with bicarbonate of soda.

To Restore Flowers To Freshness

Hold the end of the stems in the fire until they are completely charred. This may be done in the evening, and in eight hours they will be restored to vigor.

To Restore Fading Flowers

Most flowers fade within four and 24 hours after they have been placed in water, but almost all can be preserved for a much longer period, if they be in the first instance placed in warm instead of cold water. When they begin to droop, the stems should be plunged into boiling water to about one-third of their length, and by the time the water is cold, the flowers will have regained their freshness. That part which has been in the boiling water must then be cut off, and the flowers replaced in cold water.

To Take Mildew Out Of Linen

Wet the linen which contains the mildew with soft water; rub it well with white soap, then scrape some fine chalk to powder and rub it well into the linen. Lay it out on the grass in the sunshine, watching to keep it damp with soft water. Repeat the process the next day and in a few hours the mildew will entirely disappear.

To Clean Windows

1 or 2 Tb. ammonia added to a pail of water will clean windows better than soap.

To Clean Old Brass

Pour strong ammonia on the article and scrub with a brush, then rinse.

To Clean Dishcloths and Dishtowels

Put a tsp. of ammonia into the water in which these cloths are washed; rub soap on the towels. Put them in the water; let them stand half an hour or so; then rub them out, rinse and dry outdoors in the sun.

To Take Paint Out Of Clothing

Equal parts of ammonia and turpentine will take paint out of clothing, even if it be hard and dry. Saturate the spots as often as necessary, and wash out in soap suds.

To Remove Stains In Coffee and Tea Cups

Rub them with salt.

To Remove Iron Rust Or Ink Spots

Moisten the spots with salt and cream of tartar, or salt and lemon juice, exposing to full heat of the sun.

To Remove Mildew

Rub common yellow soap on the article; then salt and starch over that; rub all in will and lay in the bright sunshine.

To Remove Fruit Or Tea Stains On Table Linens

Use bicarbonate of soda in the water.

To Clean Jewelry

Put jewelry in a flannel bag with bicarbonate of soda and shake freely, or let it remain and jewelry will become bright and clean.

To Remove A Tight Ring

Thread a needle with a strong thread, pass the head of the needle with care under the ring, and pull the thread through a few inches toward the hand; wrap the long end of the thread tightly around the finger regularly to the nail to reduce its size. The lay hold of the short end and unwind it. The thread repassing against the ring, will gradually remove it from the finger. This never-failing method will remove the tightest ring without difficulty, no matter how swollen the finger may be.

To Take Out Grease

Sponge a grease spot with 4 Tbs. alcohol to one of salt.

GUIDE TO HEALING HERBS

Alfalfa

Alfalfa is a well-known herb to health-conscious consumers. It is high in nutrients, which are drawn into the plant from deep in the soil. The richest land source of trace minerals, the roots of Alfalfa plants have been known to reach as much as thirty feet deep! The leaves of the alfalfa plant are rich in minerals and nutrients, including calcium, magnesium, potassium, and carotene. They are also a source of protein, vitamin E and vitamin K. Alfalfa has been used by the Chinese since the sixth century to treat kidney stones, and to relieve fluid retention and swelling. Alfalfa nourishes the digestive, skeletal, glandular, and urinary systems. Alfalfa contains chlorophyll, which is renowned for its cleansing qualities.

Aloe Vera

Aloe vera has historically been known for assisting the functions of the gastrointestinal tract, and for its properties of soothing, cleansing and helping the body to maintain healthy tissues. This plant has a reputation of facilitating digestion, aiding blood and lymphatic circulation, as well as kidney, liver and gall bladder functions. Aloe contains at least three anti-inflammatory fatty acids that are helpful for the stomach, small intestine and colon. It naturally alkalizes digestive juices to prevent overacidity - a common cause of digestive complaints. A newly discovered compound in aloe, acemannan, is currently being studied for its ability to strengthen the immune system. Studies have shown acemannan to boost T-lymphocyte cells that aid natural resistance.

Angelica Root

Angelica nutritionally supports the digestive and respiratory systems.

Anise

Anise seeds act to remove excess mucus in the gastrointestinal area.

Barberry

Barberry nourishes the liver and gallbladder and helps the bile to flow freely. It helps remove toxins from the bowels.

Bayberry

Bayberry is an excellent blood purifier and detoxifier. It is effective for helping to stop a cold from forming if taken when the first symptoms appear.

Bdellium Gum

Bdellium gum has many positive effects on the human body. Studies show they include: lowering cholesterol levels, reducing tissue inflammation, promoting balance in the thyroid gland, and lowering body weight.

Bilberry

Bilberry (Vaccinium myrtillus) contains nutrients that protect eyes from eyestrain or fatigue, and can improve circulation to the eyes.

When British Royal Air Force pilots During World War II ate Bilberry preserves before night missions and discovered that their night vision improved afterwards, this herb was investigated and found to be very beneficial for the eyes. Bilberry works by improving the microcirculation and regeneration of retinal purple, a substance required for good eyesight. It is believed that this property is related to the high amount of proanthocyanidins, a type of flavonoid that tends to prevent capillary fragility and strengthen the capillaries which nourish the eyes.

Other properties appear to assist in thinning the blood and stimulating the release of vasodilators. Anthocyanin, a natural antioxidant, also lowers blood pressure, reduces clotting and improves blood supply to the nervous system. Anthocyanosides support and enhance the health of collagen structures in the blood vessels of the eyes, thus aiding in the development of strong healthy capillaries that can carry vital nutrients to eye muscles and nerves.

Bilberry has long been a remedy for poor vision and "night blindness." Clinical tests have indicated that oral administration of bilberry tends to improve visual accuracy in healthy people and can help those with eye disorders such as pigmentosa, retinitis, glaucoma, and myopia.

Bissy Nut

Bissy nut (Cola acuminate) has been known to help relieve inflammation in disorders such as rheumatism and gout. It also is used as a diuretic, and contains metabolism-enhancing properties.

Black Cohosh

The early Native Americans used Black Cohosh to treat snakebite and a tea from the root is reputed to soothe sore throat. They also used the root to help ease complaints associated with the skeletal system. It is a traditional approach for many gynecological topics, including menstrual cramps, labor and delivery, and menstruation. When combined with other nervine herbs, it provides excellent soothing properties. Black Cohosh also nourishes the respiratory system. Black Cohosh has traditionally been used to calm the nervous system by nourishing blood vessels, and balancing the hormones in menopausal women. Studies show it contains substances that bind to estrogen receptors. It has also been shown in lab experiments (in vitro) to inhibit microbial activity.

Black Currant Oil

Black currant oil is rich in linoleic acid and gamma-linolenic acid (GLA). This substance supports the body's manufacture of hormone-like substances known as prostaglandins which help regulate functions of the circulatory system. GLA assists the body with its energy processes and is a structural component of the brain, bone marrow, muscles and cell membranes.

Black Walnut

Black walnut hulls contain a substance which helps the body eliminate parasites. Although this is the primary purpose of this herb, it is also used for poison oak, ringworm and skin ailments. It has antifungal properties and is also said to promote bowel regularity.

Blessed Thistle

Blessed thistle acts as a general tonic to the female reproductive system, as well as helping to balance the hormones.

Blue Cohosh

Blue Cohosh nutritionally supports the female reproductive system.

Blue Vervain

Blue Vervain nourishes the digestive, nervous and respiratory systems. It helps the body maintain balance during the winter season, and fortifies it against the organisms which promote flu, coughs and colds. This herb acts as a diaphoretic, which means that it helps the body eliminate toxins through the pores by stimulating perspiration.

Burdock

Burdock is a natural blood purifier and detoxifier. It is favored for helping the body maintain healthy skin. It nourishes the urinary and respiratory systems, and also nutritionally supports joints and other skeletal tissues. It is reported to promote glandular and hormone balance, as well as remove accumulations and deposits around the joints.

Cascara Sagrada

Cascara sagrada is used to help the body relieve constipation. However, it is reputed not to be habit-forming and also nutritionally supports the stomach, liver, pancreas, and gallbladder. It is cleansing, as well as nourishing, to the colon. It is also known to assist with digestion, and help the body to eliminate worms and parasites.

Catnip

Catnip nourishes the stomach and nerves. It calms the nervous system and is used also for digestion. Catnip is also said to help ease symptoms of the flu such as nausea and diarrhea.

Cat's Claw

The highly effective properties contained in the inner bark of the cat's claw plant have demonstrated, through centuries of usage dating back to the time of the ancient Incas, to have a profound and positive influence on the body's defense system. Studies conducted since the 1970s at research clinics in Peru, Austria, Germany, England, Hungary and Italy validate the traditional usage and indicates that this herb may be beneficial in ameliorating a host of modern day afflictions which have no answers from the orthodox medical arena. It is known to help nutritionally support the body's defense, circulatory and gastrointestinal systems through its antioxidant and build properties.

Cayenne

Cayenne is a pepper well known for its benefits to the circulatory system. It aids the body to balance pressure levels and resist abnormal bleeding. Cayenne also nourishes the digestive system. This plant assists in the body's utilization of other herbs, when used in an herbal combination. When applied topically, it helps relieve minor discomfort.

Celery Seed

Celery seeds contain vitamins A, C and B-complex.

Chamomile

Chamomile soothes the nerves and stomach. It nourishes the respiratory tract and helps alleviate discomfort associated with menstrual problems.

Chickweed

Chickweed helps the body eliminate mucus and fatty plaque from the system. It nourishes the gastrointestinal areas and has soothing properties. It is a natural blood cleanser, as well as an herb that addresses fat accumulations.

Comfrey

Comfrey nourishes the pituitary gland (the master gland of the body), as well as the bones and skin. It also strengthens the respiratory system and is considered to be one of nature's great healers.

Cranberry

Cranberry contains a compound that prevents bacteria from adhering to the walls of the bladder and rest of the urinary tract. This prevents the bacteria from spreading and eventually results in the halt of infection. Using cranberry on a regular basis may help prevent the formation of kidney stones.

Cyani Flowers

Cyani flowers soothe the nervous system and exert a positive influence on tissues of the eyes.

Damiana

Damiana is known for its aphrodisiac properties, and has also been used for nervousness, weakness and exhaustion. It is said to increase sperm count in the male and to balance hormones in women.

Dandelion

Dandelion nourishes the liver and contains many vital nutrients. Dandelion root has been used traditionally to purify the blood, and to benefit the circulatory and glandular systems.

Devil's Claw

Devil's claw is an herb which has been well-known in Europe and Africa for hundreds of years and is gaining popularity in the United States and the entire North American continent. It is known for its ability to nourish the skeletal system. Studies indicate that its action is similar to cortisone. It helps the body lessen the severity of pain in joints and connective tissues.

Dong Quai

Dong quai calms the central nervous system and nourishes the brain. It also balances and strengthens the female organs and regulates their functions.

Echinacea

Modern scientific studies now validate Echinacea's traditional usage as a topical agent to help the body repair skin wounds, and internally to enhance the immune system. The active constituents in Echinacea which are thought to bolster the body's defense are known as polysaccharides. Polysaccharides stimulate the activity of macrophages, white blood cells which destroy bacteria, viruses, other foreign invaders, and even wayward cells. It also activates the body's production of interferon, a specific protein which protects cells against the invasion of viruses.

Elderberry Flowers

Elderberry flowers can help rid the body cells of toxins, increase circulation and purify the blood.

Elecampane

Elecampane is a natural expectorant and nourishes the respiratory system.

Ephedra Sinica

This Chinese herb (Ma huang) is nutritionally beneficial for fat reduction and increased energy. It facilitates energy and heat exchange for efficient metabolic function.

False Unicorn

False unicorn is considered a tonic to the reproductive organs and addresses symptoms of headaches and depression in menopausal women.

Fennel

Fennel helps detoxify and remove waste material from the body.

Fenugreek

Fenugreek has many traditional uses, including nourishing the skin, respiratory system, and the pancreas. It helps the body to expel mucus and toxins. Fenugreek dissolves fat and is high in nutrients.

Flax Seed Oil

Flax seed oil provides omega 3 (linolenic acid), omega 6 and omega 9 fatty acids. Omegas 3 and 6 benefit the cardiovascular system, as well as the immune and nervous systems. It also contains some beta carotene (approximately 4,300 IU per teaspoon) and vitamin E (appproximately 15 IU per teaspoon).

Garcinia Cambogia

Garcinia cambogia is a South Asian plant that is nutritionally beneficial in blocking the production of fats. Scientific research conducted on this herb since 1969 demonstrates that it slows the body's conversion of carbohydrates and excess calories to fat, decreasing production of harmful fats (low-density lipoproteins), promoting sustained energy levels by enhancing the body's production of glycogen, reducing the body's desire for excess food; helping to nutritionally support the metabolism and burn calories. Human studies indicate that Garcinia, also known as HCA (hydroxycitric acid) may be especially effective when combined with chromium and L-carnitine.

Garlic

Garlic provides nourishment for the circulatory, immune and urinary systems. It aids in supporting with normal circulation, nourishing stomach tissues, maintaining normal blood pressure and aids the body's natural ability to resist disease. Garlic is a natural antibiotic and fungicide.

Gentian Root

Gentian Root nourishes and strengthens the digestive system. It stimulates the appetite, nutritionally supports the liver, and nourishes the spleen, pancreas, stomach and kidneys.

Ginger

Ginger root is nourishing to the gastrointestinal system. It also helps the body to eliminate wastes through the skin. Ginger enhances circulation and acts as a catalyst for other herbs, to increase their effectiveness. It helps the body relieve congestion.

Ginkgo Biloba

Ginkgo biloba is one of the most promising and highly studied natural botanicals. Current interest in ginkgo began in the Orient, where it has long been valued for its effects on the challenges of aging. Ginkgo is effective in nutritionally supporting the body's systems, especially through its antioxidant properties. This is especially important as we grow older. Aging is a process of deterioration. The hypothesis that free radicals (reactive molecules) in the body are a direct cause of this deterioration is gaining widespread acceptance. Recently, the benefits of antioxidant vitamins in reducing free radicals in the the body have been widely published. Ginkgo is a very potent free radical scavenger. Eliminating free radicals is important in preserving youthfulness. If we slow down the deterioration of our body systems, we can enjoy fitness and vitality all through our lives.

Ginseng

Ginseng is nutritionally beneficial for the immune system and long term energy. It nourishes the circulatory system and enhances mental alertness and stamina.

Golden Seal

Golden seal is used both internally and externally to help the body fight infections with its nutritional properties. It helps the body soothe inflammations of the mucous membranes and balance their function. This herb especially nourishes the liver, glandular and respiratory systems. Golden seal helps cleanse the system of foreign organisms.

Gotu Kola

Gotu kola nourishes the nervous system, especially the brain. It is said to help improve memory and enhance vitality throughout the body. This herb is known for helping the body to balance blood pressure levels and assist in the healing of wounds. Gotu Kola is known in India as a "longevity" herb.

Hawthorn Berries

Hawthorn is traditionally known for its strong and powerful effect on the circulatory system, particularly the heart. It has been used for centuries with great success, especially in

Europe. Even today it remains a favorite among herbalists as a cardiac tonic. Hawthorn is valued for nourishing blood pressure and circulation. When used on a regular, long-term basis hawthorn exerts a continued protection to the cardiovascular system.

Hops

Hops helps the body with pain and insomnia. Hops is rich in nutrients that nourish the nervous system. The herbalist Culpeper said, "It opens obstructions of the liver and spleen, cleanses the blood, loosens the belly, cleanses the veins from gravel and provokes urine." This plant is considered both a tonic and relaxant.

Horehound Root

Horehound root is soothing to the respiratory system and is a natural expectorant.

Horsetail

Horsetail is rich in "beauty" nutrients that nourish the nails, skin, hair, bones and the body's connective tissue. It is also benefits the glands and urinary tract. Horsetail helps heal fractured bones because of its rich supply of nutrients.

Ho Shou Wu

Ho shou wu (Fo-Ti) is fabled in Asian history to restore the original color of graying hair. It nourishes the glandular, nervous, and skeletal systems. This herb is reputed to enhance the health of the liver and kidneys. The properties of Ho Shou Wu are said to be similar to Golden Seal, Chamomile and Ginseng. It is known to help improve health, stamina and resistance to diseases.

Hydrangea

Hydrangea has traditionally been used to strengthen the urinary tract and help regulate its function. This plant contains alkaloids which help soothe the body, especially in the bladder and kidney areas. Hydrangea also works like a natural inflammation reliever and cleanses the joint areas.

Hyssop

Hyssop has been used for hundreds of years as an herbal remedy for afflictions of the respiratory system. It soothes throats and nourishes the lungs.

Irish Moss

Irish moss is high in nutrients and nourishes the glandular system, lungs, and kidneys. It purifies the body's cells and strengthens the thyroid gland.

Juniper Berry

Juniper berries strengthen the urinary system and help the body eliminate excess water and toxins.

Kava Kava

Kava kava soothes the nerves.

Kelp

Kelp contains nearly thirty minerals which nourish the glands (especially the thyroid and pituitary). By enhancing the action of the glandular system, it helps balance the body's metabolism and rate at which it burns calories. Kelp, also known as seaweed, grows in the rich ocean beds, far below surface pollution levels. Because of its high nutrient content, this herb is reputedly beneficial for a wide range of applications. It is known to nourish the sensory nerves, brain membranes, also spinal cord and brain tissue. Kelp contains alginic acid which can help protect the body against the effects of radiation.

Lady Slipper

Lady slipper is a member of the orchid family. This delicate flower contains in its root many nervine properties.

Licorice

Licorice root nutritionally supports the respiratory and gastrointestinal systems, heart and spleen. This herb can soothe irritated mucous membranes and help the body get rid of unwanted mucus with its expectorant properties. Licorice Root has properties similar to cortisone and estrogen. It stimulates the adrenal glands and helps the body cope with stress.

Lobelia

Lobelia has been traditionally revered for its soothing properties that nourish the nervous system. Lobelia also enhances the function of the respiratory system and has antispasmodic effects. It has been used in preparations designed to lessen one's desire for nicotine.

Male Fern

Male fern helps the body get rid of tapeworm.

Mandrake

Mandrake works with the liver, gallbladder and all aspects of digestion. It exerts a powerful influence on the glands.

Marshmallow

Marshmallow has soothing properties and nutritionally supports the respiratory and gastrointestinal systems.

Milk Thistle

Milk thistle extract is a potent antioxidant which prevents harm from free radicals and lends nutritional support to the liver. Milk thistle seed extract contains silymarin, a unique type of flavonoid-like compound considered the active ingredient of milk thistle.

Mullein

Mullein has been referred to as a "natural wonder herb" which soothes the lungs and irritations associated with the respiratory tract. It also nourishes the lymphatic and glandular systems. Mullein can help remove mucus from the system.

Myrrh Traditionally, the properties of myrrh resin have been highly favored for soothing muscles and wounds. Myrrh nourishes mucuous membranes with its cleansing effects. The extract, when combined with water, is excellent as a comforting gargle for a scratchy throat.

Noni

The noni plant has many folk-remedy uses. It is fabled among the Polynesian peoples to especially help support the body's respiratory, immune, digestive, and structural systems.

Oatstraw

Oatstraw contains high amounts of bone-building materials.

Pan Pien Pien

Pan pien lien helps the body remove obstructions and congestion, thus strengthening and improving many areas. It nourishes and strengthens the lung areas, as well as soothing the muscles and joints.

Papaya

Papaya contains an enzyme called papain which helps the body break down protein.

Parruva Brava

Parruva brava nourishes the thermogenic processes of the body. It has been traditionally valued for its purification properties which promote perspiration.

Parsley

Parsley is valued as a blood builder, cleanser and has pressure regulating properties.

Pau d'Arco

Pau d'arco is a South American herb which helps strengthen and nourish the body's defense system. A healthy immune system is a key in fighting diseases and infections.

Passionflower

Passionflower has been used to help the body reduce anxiety, hysteria and nervousness by nourishing the nervous system. Passionflower has been traditionally used in both herbal and homeopathic medicine for pain, insomnia, nervous exhaustion, asthma and attention deficit disorder. In vitro experiments show that passicol, an alkaloid found in passionflower, kills a range of molds, yeasts, and bacteria.

Peppermint

Peppermint calms the stomach, intestinal tract, and the nervous system. It comforts the stomach and nourishes the salivary glands to help with digestion. It has astringent properties and soothes the nervous system.

Periwinkle

Periwinkle helps relieve congestion and aids in maintaining balanced circulation.

Pippali Fruit

Pippali fruit is a pepper which has been used extensively in Ayurvedic medicine to address digestive disorders and obesity.

Prickly Ash

Prickly Ash nourishes and enhances circulation throughout the entire body.

Queen of the Meadow

Queen of the Meadow is traditionally valued to help heal strains, sprains, and the associated aches. It nourishes the ligaments and tendons, and assists in restoring their normal function. It helps release inorganic deposits from the joints and tissues.

Quercetin

Quercetin has been shown to help the body defend itself against harmful microorganisms.

Raspberry Leaf

Red raspberry leaf strengthens the uterus wall and regulates menstrual flow. It nourishes the reproductive organs, especially the uterine muscles, and helps strengthen and prepare the body for childbirth. It is also highly valued for its soothing and astringent properties to the stomach and intestinal tract. Raspberry leaf is a nutrient-rich herb that helps balance the body so that diarrhea or constipation can be relieved.

Rhubarb

Rhubarb can help dissolve mucus adhering to the walls of the colon.

Safflower

The flowers of the safflower plant are used to nourish the liver, gallbladder and respiratory system. Safflower helps balance cholesterol in the body, and assists in eliminating excessive uric acid. It helps break up phlegm and soothes the digestive system.

Sage

Sage helps check excessive mucus in the body.

Sarsaparilla

Sarsaparilla contains substances which are similar to the male hormone testosterone and the female hormone progesterone. It can safely help increase the metabolic rate and balance the glandular system.

Saw Palmetto

Saw palmetto berry is said to nourish glandular tissue, and has been used by herbalists and others to nutritionally support the prostate gland.

Schizandra Chinensis

Schizandra chinensis helps the body adapt to stress and nourishes the nervous system.

Scullcap

Scullcap is one of the most powerful herbs to help you get a better night's sleep. It calms the nervous system, relaxes the muscles, and helps balance blood pressure.

Senega Root

Senega root nourishes the respiratory tract.

Senna

Senna assists in expelling waste from the intestines and kills worms.

Siberian Ginseng

Siberian ginseng nutritionally supports the glandular system. It is called an "adaptogen", which means that it helps the body adapt to any situation which normally would alter its function. Siberian Ginseng has a beneficial effect on the heart and circulation. It stimulates the entire body energy to overcome stress, fatigue, and weakness. Studies suggest that Siberian Ginseng may help reduce blood sugar levels, balance blood pressure levels, and enhance the immune system by boosting the body's production of natural killer cells.

Slippery Elm

Slippery elm can help the body eliminate mucus from the lungs and strengthen the gastrointestinal and respiratory systems. It soothes irritated tissues and helps nourish and strengthen the body.

Squaw Vine

Squaw vine strengthens the uterus, and helps relieve congestion there and in the ovaries. It may help strengthen the defense against vaginal infections.

Suma

Suma is an adaptogen herb, which means it helps the body adapt to stress, and acts as a tonic to the entire system. By enhancing the body's immune system, Suma aids in preventing free-radical damage to the body. Suma contains significant amounts of Germanium, a trace mineral which stimulates the immune system and helps promote oxygen flow to cells. It also contains "allantoin", a substance which assists in healing wounds. Some of Suma's other beneficial nutrients include vitamins, minerals, essential amino acids, and the natural plant hormones sitosterol and stigmasterol. These phytochemicals nourish the circulatory and glandular systems. The Japanese investigated Suma in trials against specific types of tumor cells. The researchers discovered that six saponins called pffaffosides A, B, C, D, E, and F are the unique chemicals present in Suma that inhibit tumor cell growth. Brazilian researchers have found that Suma is both safe and effective for altered-immune disorders.

Thyme

Thyme is known as a powerful antiseptic and a general tonic, with healing powers. It is said to be used in cases of anemia, bronchial and intestinal disturbances.

Uva Ursi

Uva ursi strengthens the urinary system and helps the body eliminate excess water.

Valerian

Valerian root nourishes the nervous system and has soothing properties. Valerian is a safe and natural sleeping aid. It helps soothe rattled nerves and assists the body in relieving insomnia. Properties of the plant have demonstrated to give calming relief to muscles, the nerves and blood vessels.

Watermelon Seeds

Watermelon seeds help the body eliminate excess water.

White Oak

White oak bark is a marvelous herb to help nourish and strengthen injured areas of the body. It has been used successfully for many applications, including fortifying blood vessels and tissues. White Oak has astringent properties, and it also soothes the throat.

White Willow

White willow benefits the stomach, kidneys, bowels, and intestines. It works like a mild and natural analgesic which is gentle on the stomach.

Wild Cherry Bark

Wild Cherry Bark is considered to be a very useful expectorant.

Wild Yam

Wild yam has many effective uses. It is known to relax the muscles and promote glandular balance in women. Wild Yam contains natural plant components known as phytochemicals which help the body balance hormone levels. Wild Yam nourishes the digestive system and the nerves.

Wood Betony

Wood betony works well for both children and adults. It is said to help migraine headaches.

Wormwood

Wormwood helps eliminate worms and parasites.

Yellow Dock Root

Yellow dock root is a bitter herb noted for its high iron content. It nourishes the skin, stimulates bile production, tones the liver and gallbladder and purifies the blood.

Yerba Santa

Yerba Santa helps the body expel mucus from the respiratory tract. It is known as a blood purifier and strengthener of the digestive system.

HERBS AND FOODS THAT MAY LEAD TO COMPLICATIONS IF YOU USE THEM WITH DRUGS

Many people have the mistaken notion that, being natural, all herbs and foods are safe. This is not so. Very often, herbs and foods may interact with medications you normally take that result in serious side reactions. It is always a good practice to tell your doctor or health practitioners what you are taking so that they can advise you of possible complications, if any. You should also keep an eye for unusual symptoms. Very often, this may foretell the symptoms of a drug interaction or more serious condition.

Experts suggest that natural does not mean it is completely safe. Everything you put in your mouth has the potential to interact with something else. The medication that is taken by mouth travels through the digestive system in much the same way as food and herbs taken orally do. So, when a drug is mixed with food or another herb, each can alter the way the body metabolizes the other. Some drugs interfere with the body's ability to absorb nutrients. Similarly, some herbs and foods can lessen or increase the impact of a drug.

As more and more people discover new herbs, there is more and more potential for the abuse of these herbs and the patients may end up with serious problems.

After attending an herb meeting a few weeks ago a person came to the speaker and told her that she had very good luck with St. John's Wort to control her depression. St. John's Wort has been shown to have great potential to control minor depression.

The National Institutes of Health is conducting a clinical study to determine the effect of St. John's Wort scientifically. This person, however, continued saying that she is now trying St. John's Wort for her OCD (Obsessive Compulsive Disorder). Now, this is getting into unproven uncharted territory. If you are taking prescription medication for this disorder, you can get into trouble due to drug interaction. As shown under the discussion on

St. John's Wort, the herb can be quite dangerous, as it acts similar to MAO inhibitors. They have severe side reactions, and if not careful, can even lead to death.

High-risk patients, such as the elderly, and patients taking three or more medications for chronic conditions, patients suffering from diabetes, hypertension, depression, high cholesterol or congestive heart failure, should be especially on the lookout for such side effects and reactions.

The following are the examples of known interaction between popular herbs, foods, and prescription and over-the-counter drugs.

Hawthorn, touted as effective in reducing angina attacks by lowering blood pressure and cholesterol levels, should never be taken with Lanoxin (digoxin), the medication prescribed for most for heart ailments. The mix can lower your heart rate too much, causing blood to pool, bringing on possible heart failure.

Ginseng, according to research, can increase blood pressure, making it dangerous for those trying to keep their blood pressure under control. Ginseng, garlic or supplements containing ginger, when taken with the blood-thinning drug, Coumadin, can cause bleeding episodes.

Coumadin is a very powerful drug that leaves little room for error, and patients taking it should never take any medication or otherwise before consulting a qualified health professional. In rare cases, ginseng may over stimulate resulting in insomnia. Consuming caffeine with ginseng increases the risk of overstimulation and gastrointestinal upset. Long tern use of ginseng may cause menstrual abnormalities and breast tenderness in some women. Ginseng is not recommended for pregnant or lactating women.

Garlic capsules combined with diabetes medication can cause a dangerous decrease in blood sugars. Some people who are sensitive to garlic may experience heartburn and flatulence. Garlic has anti-clotting properties. You should check with your doctor if you are taking anticoagulant drugs.

Goldenseal is used for coughs, stomach upsets, menstrual problems and even arthritis. However, the plant's active ingredient will raise blood pressure, complicating treatment for those taking antihypertensive medications, especially beta-blockers. For patients taking medication to control diabetes or kidney disease, this herb can cause dangerous electrolyte imbalance. High amount of consumption can lead to gastrointestinal distress and possible nervous system effects. Not recommended for pregnant or lactating women.

Feverfew, believed to be the natural remedy for migraine headaches, should never be taken with Imitrex or other migraine medications. It can result in the patient's heart rate and blood pressure to rise dangerous levels.

Guarana, an alternative remedy being used as a stimulant and diet aid, contains 3 percent to 5 percent more caffeine than a cup of coffee. So, if you are taking any medication that advises you against taking any drink with caffeine, you should avoid taking this stimulant. It may cause insomnia, trembling, anxiety, palpitations, urinary frequency, and hyperactivity. Avoid during pregnancy and lactation period. Long term use of Guarana may lead to decreased fertility, cardiovascular disease, and several forms of cancer.

Kava, a herb that has anti-anxiety, pain relieving, muscle relaxing and anticonvulsant effects, should not be taken together with substances that also act on the central nervous system, such as alcohol, barbiturates, anti depressants, and antipsychotic drugs.

St. John's Wort is a popular herb used for the treatment of mild depression. The active ingredient of St. John's Wort is hypericin. Hypericin is believed to exert a similar influence on the brain as the monoamine oxidase (MAO) inhibitors such as the one in major antidepressants. Mixing MAO inhibitors with foods high in tyramine, an amino acid, produces one of the most dramatic and dangerous food-drug interactions. Symptoms, which can occur within minutes of ingesting such foods while taking an MAO inhibitor, include rapid rise in blood pressure, a severe headache, and perhaps collapse and even death. Foods high in tyramine include aged cheese, chicken liver, Chianti (and certain other red wines), yeast extracts, bologna (and other processed meats), dried or pickled fish, legumes, soy sauce, ale, and beer.

Some patients report that Saint John's Wort caused excessive stimulation and sometimes dizziness, agitation and confusion when taken with other antidepressants or over-the-counter medications like Maximum Strength Dexatrim and Acutrim. It also caused their blood pressure to shoot up.

White Willow, an herb traditionally used for fever, headache, pain, and rheumatic complaints may lead to gastrointestinal irritation, if used for a long time. It exhibits similar reactions as aspirin (aspirin is derived from white willow). Long term use may lead to stomach ulcers.

DRUG INTERACTION WITH FOODS

Drug interaction risk isn't limited to herbal supplements. Certain foods can interact with medications.

People taking digoxin should avoid Black licorice (which contains the ingredient glycyrhizin). Together, they can produce irregular heart rhythms and cardiac arrest; licorice and diuretics will produce dangerously low potassium levels, putting a patient at risk for numbing weakness, muscle pain and even paralysis. Licorice can also interact with blood pressure medication or any calcium channel blockers.

Aged cheese (brie, parmesan, cheddar and Roquefort), fava beans, sauerkraut, Italian green beans, some beers, red wine, pepperoni and overly ripe avocados should be avoided by people taking MAO antidepressants. The interaction can cause a potentially fatal rise in blood pressure.

And because Saint Johns Wort contains the same properties as these MAO antidepressants, it stands to reason that people ingesting the herb should avoid these same foods.

Grapefruit juice interacts with calcium channel blockers (including Calan, Procardia, Nifedipine, and Verapamil), cholesterol control medications, some psychiatric medications, estrogen, oral contraceptives and many allergy medications (Seldane, Hismanal). The juice modifies the body's way of metabolizing the medication, affecting the liver's ability to work the drug through a person's system.

Orange juice shouldn't be consumed with antacids containing aluminum. The juice increases the absorption of the aluminum. Orange juice and milk should be avoided when taking antibiotics. The juice's acidity decreases the effectiveness of antibiotics, as does milk.

Milk also doesn't mix with laxatives containing bisacodyl (Correctol and Dulcolax). You might find the laxative works a little "too well" in the morning.

Large amounts of oatmeal and other high-fiber cereals should not be eaten when taking digoxin. The fiber can interfere with the absorption of the drug, making the act of swallowing the pill a waste of time.

However, don't stop eating your cereal right away, because that could cause digoxin levels in your system to soar to toxic levels. A professional should make the dietary changes after carefully examining the digoxin levels.

Leafy green vegetables, high in vitamin K, should not be taken in great quantities while taking Coumadin. These vegetables could totally negate the affects of the drug and cause blood clotting.

Caffeinated beverages and asthma drugs taken together can cause excessive excitability. Those taking Tagament (Simetidine), quinolone antibiotics (Cipro, Penetrex, Noroxin) and even oral contraceptives should be aware these drugs may cause their cup of coffee to give them more of a Java jolt than they expected.

Grilled meat can lead to problems for those on asthma medications containing theophyllines. The chemical compounds formed when meat is grilled somehow prevent this type of medication from working effectively, increasing the possibility of an unmanageable asthma attack.

Regularly consuming a diet high in fat while taking anti-inflammatory and arthritis medications can cause kidney damage and can leave the patient feeling drowsy and sedated.

Alcoholic beverages tend to increase the depressive effects of medications such as benzodiazepines, antihistamines, antidepressants, antipsychotics, muscle relaxants, narcotics, or any drug with sedative actions.

It's a good idea to not consume any alcoholic beverages, or at least scale way back, when taking prescription medications. Antioxidant and beta-carotene intensify alcohol's effect on the liver. Other commonly used over-the-counter medications can cause interaction problems also.

Aspirin can modify the effectiveness of arthritis medications, strong prescription steroids and diuretics. Combining aspirin with diabetic medications can drop blood sugars to dangerous levels. Aspirin can also cause toxicity when taken with glaucoma and anticonvulsant (anti-seizure) drugs and cause bleeding episodes when combined with a blood thinner, like Coumadin.

Acetaminophen can also cause interaction complications when overused. Heavy drinkers who take acetaminophen for hangover relief risk liver damage. Taking high doses of acetaminophen with Coumadin can cause bleeding episodes.

Antacids taken with antibiotics, heart and blood pressure or thyroid medications can decrease drug absorption by up to 90 percent.

Over-the-counter antihistamines - sold under the names Actifed, Theraflu, Dimetapp, Benadryl and Comtrex should be avoided if you are taking antianxiety or antidepressant medications.

Oral contraceptives are less effective when taken with barbiturates, antibiotics, anti-fungal or tuberculosis drugs.

Turnips contain two goitrogenic substances, progoitrin and gluconasturtin, which can interfere with the thyroid glands ability to make its hormones. Although moderate consumption of goitrogens is not a hazard for healthy people, they can promote development of a goiter (an enlarged thyroid) in persons with thyroid disease.

Tomato contains small quantities of a toxic substance known as solanine that may trigger headaches in susceptible people. They are also a relatively common cause of allergies. An unidentified substance in tomatoes and tomato-based products can cause acid reflux, leading to indigestion and heartburn. Individuals who often have digestive upsets should try eliminating tomatoes for 2 to 3 weeks to see if there is any improvement.

Strawberries, Raspberries, Spinach, and Rhubarb: These contain oxalic acid, which can aggravate kidney and bladder stones in susceptible people, and reduce body's ability to absorb iron and calcium.

Raspberries contain a natural salicylate that can cause an allergic reaction in aspirin sensitive people.

The seeds from fruits such as Apple, apricot, and Quinces contain amygdalin, a compound that turns into Hydrogen Cyanide in the stomach. Eating large amount of seeds can result in cyanide poisoning.

Potatoes: Avoid potatoes with a green tint to the skin, and remove any sprouts; they will taste bitter and may contain solanine, a toxic substance that can cause diarrhea, cramps, and fatigue.

Plums, Peaches, Apricots, and Cherries: These fruits may produce allergic reaction in individuals with confirmed allergies to apricots, almonds, peaches, and cherries. People who are allergic to aspirin may also encounter problems after they have eaten plums or peaches as they contain salicylates. The pits of plums, peaches and apricots contain a compound called amygdalin. When consumed in large amounts, amygdalin breaks down into hydrogen cyanide, a poison.

Horseradish: Very high doses of horseradish can cause vomiting or excessive sweating. Avoid if you have hypothyroidism.

Turmeric: Should be avoided by persons with symptoms from gallstones.

The drug food interaction is summarized in the table below.

Drugs	Effects and Precautions
Antibiotics	
Cephalosporins, penicillin	Take on an empty stomach to speed absorption of the drugs.
Erythromycin	Don't take with fruit juice or wine, which decrease the drug's effectiveness.

Sulfa drugs	Increase the risk of Vitamin B-12 deficiency
Tetracycline	Dairy products reduce the drug's effectiveness. Lowers Vitamin C absorption

Anticonvulsants

Dilantin, phenobarbital	Increase the risk of anemia and nerve problems due to deficiency of folalte and other B vitamins.

Antidepressants

Fluoxetine	Reduce appetite and can lead to excessive weight loss
Lithium	A low-salt diet increases the risk of lithium toxicity; excessive salt reduces the drug's efficacy
MAO Inhibitors	Foods high in tyramine (aged cheeses, processed meats, legumes, wine, beer, among others) can bring on a hypertensive crisis.
Tricyclics	Many foods, especially legumes, meat, fish, and foods high in Vitamin C, reduce absorption of the drugs.

Antihypertensives, Heart Medications

ACE inhibitors	Take on an empty stomach to improve the absorption of the drugs.
Alpha blockers	Take with liquid or food to avoid excessive drop in blood

	pressure.
Antiarrhythmic drugs	Avoid caffeine, which increases the risk of irregular heartbeat.
Beta blockers	Take on an empty stomach; food, especially meat, increases the drug's effects and can cause dizziness and low blood pressure.
Digitalis	Avoid taking with milk and high fiber foods, which reduce absorption, increases potassium loss.
Diuretics	Increase the risk of potassium deficiency.
Potassium sparing diuretics	Unless a doctor advises otherwise, don't take diuretics with potassium supplements or salt substitutes, which can cause potassium overload.
Thiazide diuretics	Increase the reaction to MSG.
Asthma Drugs	
Pseudoephedrine	Avoid caffeine, which increase feelings of anxiety and nervousness.
Theophylline	Charbroiled foods and high protein diet reduce absorption. Caffeine increases the risk of drug toxicity.
Cholesterol Lowering Drugs	
Cholestyramine	Increases the excretion of folate and vitamins A, D, E, and K.

Gemfibrozil	Avoid fatty foods, which decrease the drug's efficacy in lowering cholesterol.

Heartburn and Ulcer Medications

Antacids	Interfere with the absorption of many minerals; for maximum benefit, take medication 1 hour after eating.
Cimetidine, Fanotidine, Sucralfate	Avoid high protein foods, caffeine, and other items that increase stomach acidity.

Hormone Preparations

Oral contraceptives	Salty foods increase fluid retention. Drugs reduce the absorption of folate, vitamin B-6, and other nutrients; increase intake of foods high in these nutrients to avoid deficiencies.
Steroids	Salty foods increase fluid retention. Increase intake of foods high in calcium, vitamin K, potassium, and protein to avoid deficiencies.
Thyroid drugs	Iodine-rich foods lower the drug's efficacy.

Laxatives

Mineral Oils	Overuse can cause a deficiency of vitamins A, D, E, and K.
Painkillers	

Aspirin and stronger non-steroidal anti-inflammatory drugs	Always take with food to lower the risk of gastrointestinal irritation; avoid taking with alcohol, which increases the risk of bleeding. Frequent use of these drugs lowers the absorption of folate and vitamin C.
Codeine	Increase fiber and water intake to avoid constipation.

Sleeping Pills, Tranquilizers

Benzodiazepines	Never take with alcohol. Caffeine increases anxiety and reduce drug's effectiveness.

ABOUT THE AUTHOR

Shawna Nero Newton grew up with artistic parents: her father, Norv Nero, was a celebrated oil, watercolor, and pen and ink artist. Norv also did scrimshaw, jewelry design, and glass etching. Her mother, Lynn Nero, was an artist as well; she created impeccable needlework and cross-stitch designs. In addition, Lynn did writing of her own and outstanding publications and graphic design. In other words, there was no escaping being creative in the Nero family.

Shawna began creative writing when she was 8 years old and won awards for her short stories and poems throughout the years. She was a clothing designer for recording artists for 15 years until the writing bug struck again in 1990 along with creating web sites.

Her own interest in "historical women" and herbal remedies prompted her to research how women in the 1800's medically treated relatives and neighbors with success when professional treatment was not readily available.

Shawna completed the first manuscript for Grandma's Drugstore in 1992. During the years that followed, she continued collecting more remedies from women's' journals written in the 1800's.

Shawna resides in Avondale, Arizona with her husband, Mike, along with her "fur and feather people"; Sedona the cockatiel, Kahlua the dog, and Snickers the cat while obtaining her teaching degree.

Additional copies of this book may be purchased directly through GrandmasDrugstore.com or through Amazon.com, Lulu.com, and various retail booksellers.

Made in the USA
Middletown, DE
21 March 2019